Advance Praise for *When Baby Brings the Blues*

"*When Baby Brings the Blues* is a major triumph in breaking the silence around postpartum depression and related conditions. It is a must-read not only for women suffering from the Blues, but also their parents, families and friends."

Gideon Koren MD, FRCPC, FACMT
Director, The Motherisk Program, The Hospital for Sick Children
Professor of Pediatrics, Pharmacology, Pharmacy and Medical Genetics,
.ity of Toronto
Pro... ...n Molecular
Toxicology, University of Western Ontario

"As an obstetrician, I see women who will benefit from this book on a daily basis; as a mother, I wish this book had been available when I had my children. *When Baby Brings the Blues* provides guidance and hope for anyone who has ever struggled with postpartum depression…Dr. Dalfen illuminates the darkest hour for many women."

Isabel Blumberg, MD
Clinical Instructor, Obstetrics and Gynecology, Mount Sinai Medical Center, New York

"Dr. Dalfen simplifies and demystifies postpartum mood issues, their challenges, and their solutions. No woman should have to suffer in silence. This book is an invaluable resource for mothers and their circle of support."

Amy Sky
Singer-Songwriter, host of The Baby Hour,
mental health advocate, and postpartum depression survivor

"When the birth of a child is accompanied by anxiety and depression, women can turn to *When Baby Brings the Blues* for timely advice. Dr. Ariel Dalfen writes with compassion about the experiences of real mothers and offers practical steps towards recovery. This self-help book, which also includes a host of resources on perinatal depression and treatment options, is a 'must-read' for women and their partners coping with postpartum depression."

Shari I. Lusskin, MD
Director of Reproductive Psychiatry
New York University School of Medicine

"Integrating the most current scientific knowledge with her breadth of clinical experience and wisdom, Dr. Dalfen…provides readers with the evidence-based information essential in reducing the risks of postpartum depression and related conditions, and obtaining and providing proper care. Obstetricians, midwives and family doctors can confidently recommend this well crafted book to their patients."

Molyn Leszcz, MD, FRCPC, Psychiatrist-in-Chief, Mount Sinai Hospital, Joseph and Wolf Lebovic
Health Complex Professor of Psychiatry, University of Toronto

"*When Baby Brings the Blues* presents information about diagnoses and treatments in a clear and helpful way, as well as providing many useful hints about preventing postpartum difficulties and managing life once the baby arrives. I would recommend this book to any of my pregnant or postpartum patients."

Gail Erlick Robinson MD, D.Psych, FRCPC Director, Women's Mental Health Clinic University Health Network, Professor of Psychiatry and Obstetrics/Gynecology, University of Toronto

"Rich in practical advice about the things women can do to help themselves... *When Baby Brings the Blues* tackles the stigma and mythology head-on. It provides women with help and, importantly, hope—an essential ingredient of recovery."

David S. Goldbloom, MD, FRCPC
Senior Medical Advisor, Education & Public Affairs, Centre for Addiction and Mental Health
Professor of Psychiatry, University of Toronto
Vice Chair, Mental Health Commission of Canada

"In a society where the media still depict women with postpartum depression as 'monsters,' Dr. Dalfen has provided a welcome and overdue resource. Evidence-based, practical and above all hopeful, *When Baby Brings the Blues* assures new mothers that their ambivalence, anxiety and depression are medical problems with effective solutions. Best of all—Dr. Dalfen gives these women a path to wellness."

Maureen Taylor
Former National Medical Reporter, CBC News
Physician Assistant Student, McMaster University

"This book is a must-read for women who are suffering from postpartum depression..."

Adrienne Einarson, RN
Assistant Director
The Motherisk Program, The Hospital for Sick Children

"Ariel Dalfen counters the all-too-pervasive myths about postpartum depression and anxiety by offering her readers a compelling mix of reassuring facts and compassionate wisdom. The highlight of this important book is a chapter which gets inside the heads of the new mother and her partner. This section of the book will prove invaluable to new parents who are discovering how painfully difficult it can be to find the words to express to one another what they are feeling about the unchartered territory that they have ventured into as a couple."

Ann Douglas, bestselling author, The Mother of All Pregnancy Books

"Those who are at risk or are sufferers of postpartum depression will find this book to be a priceless resource."

Dr. Shaila Misri, Director, Reproductive Mental Health Program,
BC Women's/St Paul's Hospital

When Baby Brings the Blues
Solutions for Postpartum Depresssion

Dr. Ariel Dalfen M.D.

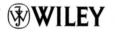

WILEY

John Wiley & Sons Canada, Ltd.

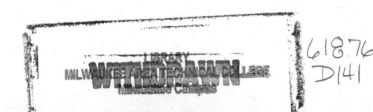

Library and Archives Canada Cataloguing in Publication Data
Dalfen, Ariel
When baby brings the blues : Solutions for postpartum depression / Ariel
Dalfen.
Includes index.
ISBN 978-0-470-15421-2
Postpartum depression—Treatment. 2. Postpartum depression—Popular
works. I. Title.
RG852.D34 2008   618.7'6   C2008-905757-0

Production Credits
Cover: Ian Koo
Interior text design and Typesetting: Michael Chan
Printer: Friesens

John Wiley & Sons Canada, Ltd.
6045 Freemont Blvd.
Mississauga, Ontario
L5R 4J3

Printed in Canada

1 2 3 4 5 FP 13 12 11 10 09

To Jed

*

To my Girls
Lela and Liv

*

To my Women
Alyce and Fay (may their memories be blessed),
Susannah, Deborah

*

To my Dad

*

To all the women who I have seen who have
struggled and overcome.

Quick Reference of Important Information, Tables and Checklists

Introduction

Did you know that all over the world, postpartum depression (PPD) and anxiety (PPA) disorders affect a full fifteen to twenty percent of new mothers? That is a staggering statistic. It is particularly disturbing that these illnesses have, until recently, received little attention from the medical profession, and limited accurate media exposure and social awareness. Because PPD and PPA impact us and our families at one of the most pivotal times of life, it is vital that we learn how to recognize and treat them. During this precious phase, we need to be healthy. We need the strength to care for ourselves, to learn how to be mothers, to connect in new ways with our partners, and of course, to care for our little babies. These are huge, wonderful tasks. But, when you are experiencing PPD or PPA, your ability to nurture yourself and your growing family is compromised—sometimes severely.

But this does not have to be the case. Both PPD and PPA are eminently treatable illnesses. We now know that there are excellent, fast-acting solutions that will help you feel well. In this book I will explain the many options available to you, and walk you through the step-by-step creation of your own, individual treatment plan. I will show you how to address your suffering head on, and what you can do about it.

Whether you are planning to get pregnant and are worried, already pregnant and are feeling badly, or if you suspect you might have PPD or PPA, there is something in this book that can help you now. If you have not yet had a baby, being aware of your risks goes a long way towards minimizing your chances of developing postpartum problems. And if you suspect you are already suffering, you need to know how to enhance the healing process, and how to get safe and successful treatment as rapidly as possible.

Unfortunately, much misinformation exists about post-partum mental health issues. This misinformation may be stopping you from realizing that you are suffering in the first place, or it may make you fearful of telling anyone about how you feel. In this book, I will address these myths and give you the most up-to-date and evidence-based information to help you understand the reality of PPD and PPA, and show you how to help yourself though this time, as well as how to find good professional help.

As I sat down one day to work on this book, my three-year-old daughter came rambling into the study. She asked me what I was doing and I told her I was writing a book. Not surprisingly, she said "Why?" I told her that I was writing a book because I really want to help new mothers feel better. This is true, but the full truth goes deeper. I am writing this book because so many women suffer needlessly, and silently. The real tragedy of PPD and PPA is that far too many new mothers go untreated; these illnesses are wonderfully responsive to a wide array of treatments—but only if those treatments are known about, understood, and made widely available.

As a psychiatrist who sees hundreds of pregnant women and new moms every year, I have become intimately familiar with the ravages of depression or anxiety at this central moment in a woman's life. But the story does not stop there; I have also been involved with the recovery of so many women. And this is what I want to share with you in this book.

If there is any time in your life to step forward and to take control of your health and well being, it is now. The costs of not getting better from PPD and PPA are just too high. You, your family, and your baby will all benefit tremendously from your recovery—"the real you" will return. You will feel that you can be there for yourself and for your baby, and you will be able to experience the full range of feelings that accompany being a new mom. You will be able to feel happiness in your life and experience the deepening connection to your partner, and to your baby.

As the wise Helen Keller once said: "Although the world is very full of suffering, it is also full of the overcoming of it."

Chapter 1
The Myths and Realities of Postpartum Mental Illness

Motherhood is surrounded by myths. There are myths about what it takes to be a good mother, about how to ensure your child thrives, about what material things you need, and about how a good mother should think, feel and act so that her child is successful and happy.

Myths about depression also abound: there are myths that depressed people are weak and lazy, that depression is not really an illness but an attitude problem, and that there must be something wrong with your personality if you suffer from depression or anxiety, to name just three.

When depression or severe anxiety affects new moms, the myths become overwhelming! Katie is a 33-year-old new mother whom I recently saw for PPD. When she first came to see me, she was deeply ashamed that she had to come for help with depression at what was supposed to be the happiest time of her life. While she was waiting in the hallway outside my office, which is near a busy obstetrics department, she felt that all the happy pregnant women were looking at her with disdain. She thought everyone was eyeing her, staring at the sign above her head that says "Mental Health Services" and judging her for being a bad mother. "Not only am I damaging my baby from the start because I'm depressed, but I must be a horrible person who is not cut out for motherhood," she told me. When we developed a treatment plan to address Katie's depression, she was amazed at how quickly she felt better. Katie realized that her misconceptions about depression, and what it meant about her as a mother, had been holding her back from getting the help she needed. She also learned that many other women also have postpartum depression or anxiety and that she is not alone.

The myths about postpartum depression are very damaging. They cause women to feel like bad mothers and to think that something is wrong with them. When these myths become too powerful, they stop you from acknowledging that you are having a hard time and isolate you with your sadness. They make you feel like something is wrong with you and that it can't be fixed. Rather than realizing that you are suffering from an actual medical problem that has a cure, the myths and misconceptions prevent you from accessing high-quality medical care and making easy, helpful changes on your own. The longer you suffer, the worse your depression becomes and the less likely you are to enjoy motherhood and bond with your little one.

There are five main myths about PPD that stop women from getting the help they need and deserve.

Let's break down each of these myths, once and for all. This will pave the way for you to recognize that you are suffering with a very treatable problem, access help, and have a happy and healthy relationship with your new baby.

"Feeling Badly Is a Normal Part of Being a New Mother"

Suzanne came to see me when she was two months postpartum. She had had an uncomplicated pregnancy and an easy labor and delivery. Then, about two weeks after her daughter was born, her husband went back to work and things began to change. She felt sad, especially now that she was alone with her daughter, and that sadness quickly grew into several episodes of crying every day. Having a baby felt like a big mistake, especially since she had been at the peak of her career.

It became harder and harder to get out of the house with the baby, and besides, she felt too exhausted to socialize or "put on a happy face." She also found that she was having trouble sleeping at night when her baby finally settled down. At nighttime she was besieged by thoughts of how she was not doing enough and not being a good enough mom. "Am I intellectually stimulating the baby enough? I should have taken her outside this afternoon. I'll have to try to do more tomorrow…." Her mind went on and on: "I'm not keeping the house clean enough. My body doesn't look thin enough…." Eventually she felt depressed every day, and her sleep got worse and worse. After about a month, Suzanne found that she really did not enjoy anything in her daily life. Laughing and taking pleasure in things that she once enjoyed was impossible, and small, daily decisions were difficult to make. When I asked Suzanne why she had let her suffering continue for so long, she was shocked by the question. She said that as a new mom she thought she was "just hormonal, and *supposed* to feel exhausted, depressed, and tormented."

Cindy gave birth to a baby who was "difficult" by all accounts. He didn't sleep for more than two hours at a time for the first six months of his life. As the sleepless weeks and months wore on, Cindy became increasingly despondent. She cried a lot and lost her appetite. She finally broke down and told her mother and sister that she was feeling overwhelmed and sad. Rather than offer her comfort and support, they simply said "Welcome to motherhood." They told her that being a mother is hard work and she should expect to feel tired at times. What else was there but to endure? So, she continued to feel drained, increasingly depressed, and miserable. Finally, she came to see me and we swiftly turned her depression around.

Suzanne and Cindy are not alone in not knowing where the challenges of motherhood end and depression begins. It does not help that those around us may not be aware either. What is the boundary between a normal adjustment to a new phase of life and PPD? We all expect motherhood to be a challenge (and it never disappoints on that front!), complete with lack of sleep, fatigue, "baby brain," and, yes, discouraging thoughts about this new role. It *can* be confusing for new moms to distinguish the symptoms of depression because many of them mimic what every new mom will experience. However, being tired, occasionally overwhelmed, daunted, and even exasperated are not the same as being depressed.

Having a baby should not leave you feeling that you cannot settle down and turn your worried mind off. It should not leave you feeling full of regret and remorse for weeks or months on end. It should not leave you feeling miserable or consistently anxious and unsettled. In the chapters ahead, you will learn more about the differences between the "normal" but hard adjustment to becoming a mother and clinical depression. You will learn about the very real and specific symptoms of depression and what to do if you have them. For now, please realize that although the early days of mothering can be tough, they should not be devastating.

Having a baby offers you the opportunity to assess and reassess the meaning of your life, your identity, your life's goals, your relationships, how you spend your time, and what your priorities are. It is normal to occasionally miss your pre-baby life or to wish that certain things about being a mother were easier. But if you are feeling sad, excessively worried, unable to enjoy life, wishing you could escape or end your life, and are unable to eat or sleep for an ongoing period of time, this is *not* normal motherhood, and you do not need to continue to feel this way. Lasting misery usually means that PPD is lurking. The sooner you recognize your symptoms, the sooner you can get started on feeling better, so don't despair, read on.

"If I Tell Anyone How I'm Feeling, They Will Take My Baby Away"

Andrea was a 25-year-old new mother. In the four months since her son was born, she had been crying every day and feeling overwhelmed and very sad. She was dragging herself around and felt that she was not doing a good job as a mother. When I saw Andrea, after she had made and canceled a few appointments with me, I asked her why she had been reluctant to seek help when it was clear that her condition was worsening and she was finding it progressively more difficult to take care of herself and her baby. She said, "I was afraid I would be labeled an unfit mother and that my son would be taken away from me." Andrea also admitted to me that her husband told her to keep her feelings to herself because he, too, was scared that if anyone knew the truth about how she was doing, they would no longer be allowed to parent the baby.

Mary gave birth to a healthy baby boy when she was 33 years old. Her pregnancy went smoothly and she was excited to become a mother. Mary had always been a bit of a worrier, but her anxiety skyrocketed as soon as her son was born. She constantly felt on edge. A few days after coming home from the hospital, Mary began to have scary thoughts about smothering her son with a pillow. These thoughts would suddenly intrude into her mind and she would get very anxious about having them. Obviously, these thoughts were incredibly frightening. She didn't really want to harm her son, and became terrified about being alone with her baby. She would not stay home alone and hid all the pillows in the house. Mary was terrified that if she told anyone about her thoughts and feelings, child-protection services would take away her son. Because Mary was so fearful about revealing her scary thoughts, she continued to suffer silently for many months. Her overwhelming and anxious feelings persisted and she became increasingly depressed. She was unable to enjoy the first six months of her son's life.

The idea that some official, external force will step in and take away your baby is one of the scariest, most powerful myths for women suffering from PPD. When women are suffering from PPD and have intrusive, unwanted thoughts about harming their babies or surprisingly negative feelings toward the baby they longed for, it is extremely frightening. If you have these thoughts and feelings, you may feel very scared about your capacity to mother and worry about your state of mind. We will talk in detail about scary thoughts, what they really mean, and how to handle them in the chapters to come. Being depressed, having scary thoughts, feeling alone or frustrated, or wanting to go back to your old life are unsettling feelings, but none of these result in children being removed from their mother's care. Babies are not taken away from moms simply because the mothers have PPD. Child-protection services are called to help only when a baby is at risk of harm or neglect.

If you are a serious drug addict, have a major psychotic illness, or a long criminal history or a partner with similar problems, child-protection services may step in because you may be unable to care for your baby under these circumstances in which your child's welfare and safety may be at risk.

Many women who have postpartum depression and postpartum anxiety problems get very anxious about "the authorities" being called. In fact, reaching out for help shows tremendous strength. This is viewed very positively by health care providers. If you know you are having trouble as a new mother and you try to get help, this is a *very* good thing. It shows you have insight into your situation and are trying to get better. It does not mean that you are an unsafe mother. Quite the opposite!

The power of the myth that "my baby will be taken away from me" prevented Andrea and Mary from talking to professionals for a long time, but they finally broke their silence, and learned that their feelings were common. When that happened, not only were they reassured that they had done the right thing, but their depression and anxiety symptoms improved with treatment and they were able to deepen their bonds with their new babies.

"I Should Just Pull Myself up by My Bootstraps"

Lisa came into my office crying three weeks after she had her first baby. She felt she could not cope with her new baby and she spent her days wishing she could hide under her covers and run away. To make matters worse, when she told her husband how she was feeling, he just didn't get it. He was a smart and well-educated guy, but all he would say to her was: "Just get over it. Pull yourself together." Of course, this made her feel like even more of a failure and incompetent as a mother. Lisa's husband finally agreed to come to one of our appointments and I explained to him that PPD is a real illness that requires real treatments and time to heal. With her husband's improved understanding, empathy, and support, Lisa not only got over her PPD, but their relationship became much stronger in the process.

The reality is that depression is a biological illness that has real and demonstrable brain and body changes. It does not reflect a weak character or a flawed personality. Sophisticated brain-imaging techniques have shown that someone who is depressed has actual significant changes going on in the brain. Depressed brains have different amounts of neurotransmitters, distinct levels and patterns of activity, and altered brain structures compared to non-depressed brains. Although these advanced scientific technologies are not widely used for the diagnosis of depression, the brain changes are well documented and highly accepted among health care professionals.

Often people who have depression are told or believe that they don't *really* have an illness that needs to be treated, but that depression is "an attitude problem." Patient after patient, like Lisa, tell me that their partner, family, and friends tell them to just pull themselves together. Many depressed people are told that they will get better if only they ignore their symptoms, or pray more, or change their diet, or just exercise. For some reason, the validity of depression as a genuine medical problem seems to be up for debate in certain circles.

Wouldn't it be nice if it was that easy to get over depression? Obviously, the "just get over it" myth is detrimental to people who have been struck by this nasty illness. This myth makes people who are suffering from depression feel like they are crazy and that they must really be weak since they can't fight this alone. Because of this myth, people who are depressed are less likely to tell others what they feel, and less likely to get help for fear of being criticized or scolded.

Not only are you feeling weak that you have depression but you are also probably feeling badly that you are experiencing this problem at a time in life when you expected so much joy.

The fact is that women who seek help for PPD get better. There is a very high rate of recovery for PPD, and most women fully recover quickly.

"If I Feel This Badly, I Am Not Meant to Be a Mother and I Am a Bad Mother"

Felicia was a 36-year-old mother of a new baby girl. She had been so excited to have a baby and had imagined loving every minute of motherhood. However, the reality did not live up to her fantasy. Her baby was colicky and kept Felicia up through the night for weeks on end. "Tired to the bone," was how she described her existence. Not only did Felicia feel exhausted, but she also felt deep regret and profound guilt about making such a drastic "mistake." She began to resent her baby and to wish that she had never become pregnant. "I miss my life with my husband and I miss my freedom," she told me when I saw her for depression. Because she felt "pummeled" by motherhood, she felt that she should never have had a child in the first place. "No woman who is feeling this badly and is this angry can possibly be a good mother," Felicia said through her tears.

Donna had a baby girl at age 30. She had wanted to get pregnant and was looking forward to becoming a mother. However, once Donna's daughter was born, she was not so sure that "the motherhood thing" was for her. She found it hard to spend all her time with her baby and got "desperately bored" of endless hours of feeding, diaper changing, watching the baby on a play mat, and talking with other new mothers about dirty diapers. She felt very alone whenever she went to new-mothers' groups because it seemed as if all of the other mothers were blissful in their new roles. "Something must be wrong with *me*," thought Donna. She felt ashamed that she was not enjoying being a mother as much as other women seemed to. Her shame prevented her from telling anyone how she was feeling, and she was convinced that she was "thoroughly inadequate" as a mother.

Being a new mother is a tremendous amount of work at the best of times, but beware of drawing the conclusion that you should not be a mother if you haven't immediately adapted to the job. This is a hard job! Just because you are feeling depressed or anxious doesn't meant you shouldn't be a mother. Depression is a real illness. Imagine how ridiculous it would sound if a woman who developed postpartum thyroid problems decided that her thyroid problems (or her need for help with her thyroid disorder) are proof that she should not be a mother. Unfortunately, depression affects how we think and feel about ourselves and clouds our good judgment, so it is easy for new moms who are depressed to buy into the myth that they should never have started down this road in the first place.

Donna had relatively minor depression and so we focused her recovery plan on dealing with issues adjusting to her role as a mother. Talk therapy really helped Donna not to compare herself to other moms and to find her own stride.

Felicia and I created a treatment plan she was comfortable with for her sleeplessness and depression, and she went on to really enjoy parenting. In fact, once she got some sleep and recovered from depression, she was able to reflect on the major changes in her life and see not only what she had lost, but also the wonderful things she had gained. By the end of the first year after her daughter's birth, she was so comfortable being a mother it wouldn't have occurred to her to think about whether or not she *should* be a mom: She just was one.

"There Are No Safe Treatments, So Why Bother Getting Help?"

Sara had a long history of depression that dated back to her teenage years. She was treated successfully in the past with antidepressant medication. However, prior to getting pregnant at age 28, she saw some news stories about the dangers of antidepressants during pregnancy. She followed up by doing extensive Internet searches through which she found lots of contradictory information. The more she searched online and the more opinions she read about in chat groups, the more confused she became, so Sara decided to stop taking her medication when she got pregnant. Unfortunately, after having her baby, Sara developed postpartum depression. When she went to see her physician, he told her that no anti-depressants were safe to take while she was breastfeeding, so she would just have to wait it out. Finally, after her husband

and mother did some research and got a referral for Sara, she came to see me. She was discouraged about the prospect of getting help after being bombarded with so much negative and confusing information. I encouraged Sara to print out information that she found online and wanted to understand. We went through her pages of questions and I addressed her concerns directly.

In our increasingly Internet-savvy culture, many patients come to see me after they have already consulted with "Dr. Google." The vast majority of people regularly use the Internet and most use it as their number one source of health information. Chances are you have gone online and already diagnosed yourself as having PPD. (As you read on in this book, you will find useful and accurate tools for understanding and diagnosing your own symptoms.) You may have also been frightened by uninformed physicians, media sources, or skeptical relatives that psychiatric treatments are ineffective and that no treatments are compatible with breastfeeding. Or, you may have spoken to people who don't "believe" in psychiatry or that any psychological treatments can be helpful. Then, like many new moms, you might conclude that since there are no effective treatments for postpartum mental issues, there is no point in getting professional help.

The reality is quite the opposite. First, it is essential to realize that there are numerous safe and effective treatments for postpartum depression. Medication may be necessary in some cases of PPD. However, talk therapy, support groups, simple changes to your sleep routine and calling on your support system to kick into action may be where your treatment starts and ends. Second, if you do require medication, there is high-quality scientific research that has demonstrated the safety of many medications during pregnancy and while breastfeeding.

Later I will go into lots of detail about what is available and what your options are based on the very latest research. For now, the most important thing for you to know is that there is help and support available from professionals, and there are many important things you can do to help yourself. You will be amazed at how much better you can feel and how you can actually love and embrace your baby as you had hoped to do in the first place.

I hope by now I have busted the myths that stop women from addressing their postpartum problems and seeking help when they need it. Later on in this book you will learn ways you can help yourself get over PPD, and how to find the right kind of professional help to help you end your suffering.

For now, you can start your healing process by ignoring the myths that surround PPD and knowing the realities about this common and eminently treatable problem.

Start feeling better by knowing the truth about PPD:

The Truth About PPD

1. It is not normal to feel down for a long time or continuously sad after you have a baby.

2. Having PPD is not a reason for anyone to take your child from you.

3. Depression is a real illness and you are really suffering. You are not a weak or lazy person.

4. Being depressed may make you think you are an inadequate mother and may make it hard for you to enjoy motherhood, but you will see the entire experience in a different light once you feel better.

5. There are excellent, safe, and effective treatments that can and will help you feel better.

Chapter 2

Are You at Risk?

Women come to see me for two main reasons: First, there are those who are pregnant or are planning to get pregnant and suspect that they will get PPD. Then there are those who are already suffering and are trying to get their lives back on track. The first consideration is a general overview, which includes such things as past experiences and illnesses, family life, and current relationships. However, there are also very specific things that can indicate whether or not someone is at risk of PPD.

Thanks to good medical research, we know quite a bit about the major risk factors for PPD, as well as for other postpartum emotional problems, including postpartum anxiety disorders (PPA) and postpartum psychosis (PPP), so we can begin to answer the essential questions: "Will you get PPD?" and "Why do you have PPD?"

You won't be surprised to know that the answers are not always totally straightforward. However, there are several proven factors that put a woman at risk. If you have just had a baby or will soon give birth, you need to know what these are. Knowing about these risk factors is an essential step toward preventing PPD.

If you are worried that you are at high risk for postpartum mental health problems, knowing your risk means that you and your partner can be prepared. You can plan ahead to minimize some of your risks, and get your supports lined up and your treatment team ready. With a lot of knowledge and a little planning, you can be well on the road toward a healthy and happy postpartum experience. By knowing and minimizing the issues that may trigger a postpartum problem for you, you can do a lot to keep a crisis at bay.

If you think you may be suffering from PPD already, this chapter will help you learn about what may have caused your illness this time, and to understand some of the stressors in your life that are perpetuating the problems. Part of getting better is learning how to address and change the things in your life that are creating or worsening your depression and anxiety. The sooner you are aware that you have PPD and identify the triggers, the more quickly you can address them and the sooner you will feel better.

> By understanding the risk factors of PPD, you can lower your chances of experiencing it.

Once you know more about your own illness and your personal risk factors, you will be able to discuss these things with your health care provider and get the appropriate treatment you need to address your particular set of circumstances.

Unfortunately, medical science in this area has not evolved to the point where we can isolate a root cause of PPD or do a specific test to determine exactly whether or not you will experience PPD. Instead, like most other psychiatric illnesses, PPD is best understood through what is called the bio-psycho-social model. This model takes into account your personal biological risk factors—which include your genetics and your physical brain and body—as well as your psychological and social risk factors. When we put all of your specific risks together, we can create an in-depth explanation about your level of risk and also understand why you may have developed PPD now.

> PPD is a complex illness with biological, psychological, and social causes.

Even though you cannot change some of your risk factors, such as your past history or your biology, you will see that many of the risk factors have to do with areas of your life over which you have quite a bit of control. This is good news! And even if you have several risk factors at once, that is okay. Even this does not mean that PPD is inevitable. Believe it or not, there are numerous ways to minimize the seemingly unchangeable risks. I will help you learn how to do this. But now, knowing which risk factors most apply to you is the first step in putting together your wellness plan or recovery program for the postpartum period. As the wise Sir Francis Bacon once said, "Knowledge is power."

> You can control many of the things that put you at risk for PPD.

The First Layer of Risk

All women experience significant hormonal changes from pregnancy and delivery. When you are pregnant, your levels of estrogen and progesterone rise steadily throughout pregnancy. When you deliver your baby, these hormones drop dramatically.

The female hormones estrogen and progesterone interact with the brain chemicals that control our moods, particularly serotonin. Although the precise nature of this relationship is yet to be determined, there does appear to be a very strong link between hormones, moods, and behavior. Given this relationship, it makes sense that striking changes in hormone levels make a woman who has recently had a baby vulnerable to mood changes.

The question is, if all childbearing women undergo similar hormonal changes, why don't they all develop PPD?

In addition to the extensive biological changes related to having a baby, it seems that you need to have a combination of other risks to get PPD. Other physical, genetic, psychological, or social issues interact with the hormonal fluctuations, causing the illness to manifest itself. It is as if all women have the first layer of risk by virtue of having a baby, but the balance is tipped by other factors. So to evaluate your own risk of PPD, or to gain a better understanding of why you may have developed PPD, let's talk about other risk factors in some detail.

Biological Risk Factors

These risks are due to physical, chemical, or hormonal changes in your brain or your body.

Depression or Anxiety During Pregnancy

One of the strongest risk factors for developing PPD is having symptoms of depression or anxiety during pregnancy. In fact, women who are depressed during pregnancy have a 50 percent chance of having PPD.

Although this statistic may sound scary, remember that even if your risk is 50 percent, you are still just as likely not to have PPD as to have it, without doing a thing. But why take the chance to doing nothing? There is so much you can do to protect and prepare yourself. Depression and anxiety during pregnancy are very treatable. We will talk all about this in more detail in the pages ahead.

> If you are depressed or anxious when you pregnant, get help now to lower your risk of PPD.

Personal and Family History of Mental Illness

If you have suffered from depression, bipolar disorder, or an anxiety disorder in the past, you are at higher risk of developing PPD. At this stressful time in your life, another episode can occur. About a quarter of all women who have experienced depression and anxiety, and half of women who have had bipolar disorder, will develop postpartum depression or a postpartum anxiety disorder, such as panic disorder, obsessive-compulsive disorder or generalized anxiety disorder. Women who have had bipolar disorder are 25–30 percent more likely to develop postpartum psychosis, which we will describe later. Again, women who have never had mental illness have a 15–20 percent chance of having PPD.

Women who have a family member who has had a mental disorder are also at increased risk of PPD. This is particularly true if your relative is your parent or sibling. The more family members who have mental illness, the higher the risk of PPD. If your mother or sister had PPD, this also increases your risk.

History of Hormone-Related Mood Changes

Many women with PPD have had mood changes or increased anxiety in the weeks before they menstruate. These symptoms may not have been severe enough to require medical attention, but they are upsetting, recognizable, and memorable.

For women who have had a low mood and feel badly before their periods, premenstrual syndrome (PMS) is commonly diagnosed. For those women who are debilitated cycle after cycle by depression, the more serious premenstrual dysphoric disorder (PMDD) is diagnosed. It seems that women who have a history of PMS or PMDD are more likely to develop PPD.

Women who have a history of developing depression when they have taken oral contraceptives or fertility drugs, such as Clomid, also appear to be at increased risk of developing PPD. For these women, changing hormone levels seem to have a negative impact on their mood and anxiety levels.

Thyroid Disorder

Thyroid problems commonly occur in women. The thyroid is a little gland at the base of the neck that secretes hormones. These hormones play a role in regulating almost all bodily functions, including temperature regulation, moods, weight, energy levels, and food metabolism, to name a few.

In the postpartum period, about 5 percent of new moms develop a condition called postpartum thyroiditis. This may occur in women who did not have obvious thyroid disease before pregnancy, but pregnancy and delivery unmask the problem. The symptoms of postpartum thyroiditis are fatigue, moodiness, heart palpitations, and sometimes an enlarged thyroid gland. Sound like familiar symptoms? Postpartum thyroiditis often looks and feels like depression and what women associate as the feelings of being a new mom. As a result, it is underdiagnosed.

Often postpartum thyroiditis develops into hypothyroidism, which means that the body continues to produce too little thyroid hormone. The symptoms of hypothyroidism can also mimic those of depression: low mood, fatigue, lethargy, and irritability. Although postpartum hypothyroidism might resolve on its own, for 25–50 percent of women, hypothyroidism becomes an ongoing condition that requires monitoring and treatment.

> If you are feeling down, fatigued, lethargic, and irritable, ask your doctor to check your thyroid.

Psychological Risk Factors

In this category are the risks related to your personality or coping style, or other factors that reflect how you may think, feel, and view the world.

Negative Thinking Patterns

Anna came to see me when she had a 10-week-old baby and was feeling very frustrated and upset. She said that whenever she tried to put her new daughter to sleep and the baby would not settle down immediately, she would call herself "a failure as a mother." She would decide in that moment that she was "not cut out to be a mother." Whenever her baby did not behave as she expected or desired, Anna would jump to the conclusion that she herself was at fault. Of course, after criticizing herself for 10 weeks, she began to feel depressed. Rather than assessing the situation in a balanced and reasonable way, such as thinking that perhaps her baby was not yet tired, or that babies often cry when they are soothing themselves to sleep, Anna quickly blamed herself and got into a downward spiral of negative emotions.

Anna's experience illustrates a negative pattern of thinking that many women get caught up in called "personalization." This occurs when someone interprets a difficult situation (about motherhood or anything else) as being her own fault and a reflection of her inadequacies.

Another common negative thinking pattern is "all or nothing thinking." Melissa was a new mother who felt down because she felt that she was not bonding with her new son. Playing and talking with her baby felt uncomfortable and awkward. She just could not follow what the baby books recommended. Worries about not connecting with her son and stunting his social development consumed Melissa. She felt that her efforts were "totally useless" and that she was "failing" her son. If she was not the "perfect mother," she would be a "total disaster."

When Melissa and I examined what she was doing with her son and how she was relating to him, it seemed that she was actually doing all the right things. She was not giving herself credit for what she was doing and was instead thinking that she was doing everything wrong.

The words "always" or "never" frequently reflect negative thinking and self-defeating cognitive patterns that can lead to depression and anxiety.

> Listen to your mind: If you find yourself frequently using words like "always" or "never," you may have an overly negative thinking pattern.

We all have unhelpful thought patterns and reactions at some times, but those who react this way much of the time are at higher risk of having postpartum depression and anxiety problems. New moms who are accustomed to using negative thinking patterns are inclined to interpret a situation in a way that makes them feel badly and very frustrated. When you view the world, a situation, or yourself in a pessimistic way, of course this can, and often does, lead to depression. It is important to realize that these negative thinking styles are only *interpretations* of a situation and do not reflect the situation itself. Later in the book I will show you some great ways to reprogram this automatic response.

The Worriers and the Perfectionists

Our personalities are made up of our emotional and behavioral responses to the world. Though it seems that there are as many personalities as there are people, our own personalities are generally constant and quite predictable, and they shape the way we deal with situations, new and old.

There are certain personality traits that seem to put women at higher risk of developing PPD. Women with particularly anxious and perfectionist personality traits are at moderate risk of developing PPD.

Women who are very anxious or neurotic tend to worry a lot about everything, and are easily upset and overwhelmed. They may worry about their baby's health and well-being, about their capacity to parent, or about the transition back to work. Having a child is difficult for all women, but if you are a worrier by nature, this stage in life will provide endless fodder to fuel your anxious mind. When a person with a neurotic personality encounters this already challenging life experience, she can easily feel barraged by the many new things to think about and deal with. Women who tend to be big worriers not only worry about every little change they see in their baby's behavior or habits, but they also worry that they cannot cope with the new situations that arise. The high degree of worry and uncertainty can lead to postpartum depression and anxiety.

For women who have a history of intense fears and worries about getting sick or having a terrible illness, having a newborn can be particularly challenging. It seems that many women with these types of anxieties grew up in families where they had to cope with the sickness of a parent or a sibling at a very young age. Illness was a big part of their childhood and the threat of death lurked. When these women have babies of their own, they tend to be very anxious about every little sign of sickness a baby may have. Of course, it is always upsetting if your baby seems unwell, but for new moms who are health worriers, the worry can be excessive and uncontrollable, and it can lead to postpartum anxiety or depression.

Perfectionists also have a hard time as new mothers. For women who are accustomed to having everything in life well organized, tidy, and perfectly done, having a child can be very unsettling and tremendously overwhelming. There is no such thing as the perfect baby who will comply with the rules and timing that a woman with perfectionist traits is accustomed to. Perfectionism can be a valuable quality that can help you to get ahead in life and in your career. It has probably helped you to stay organized and to complete tasks effectively. But if you are used to feeling good only when everything is done "just so," then having a baby can throw you for a loop. It is impossible to be a perfect mother and to have a perfect baby who will fall in line. This can be hard for some women to handle: It is unsettling when you cannot use your well-honed coping skills in a given situation. Because perfectionists' ways of coping in the world (which served them well up until now) suddenly seem to make matters worse, they can be at higher risk for feeling out of control and eventually depressed or highly anxious.

In the chapters ahead, you will learn what to do if you are a big worrier or a practiced perfectionist.

History of Abuse or Conflict with Parents

Some women who have had difficult relationships with their parents may be at increased risk of developing PPD. Having a child of your own can certainly raise issues about your childhood experiences and problems. It can remind us about the difficulties we may have had as a child, such as being abused or mistreated or feeling neglected. Nearly everyone at some point vows not to repeat their parents' mistakes, but for women who were neglected or abused, this fear is amplified. They often feel destined to repeat those same mistakes. They worry that they will not be able to avoid being abusive because they were never shown another way of raising a child. The fear of repeating the past is constant and very stressful, and can contribute to PPD. (Remember, you don't have to have a perfect past and perfect parents to be a good parent and to avoid PPD.)

Many women find that when they have a baby, they experience a strong desire to turn to their own mothers for support. When women who have had or continue to have a conflicted relationship with their parents find them unavailable for either emotional or practical support, it can be incredibly painful.

Farrah was a 38-year-old woman who came to see me after the birth of her second son. Her own parents were strict disciplinarians who were not particularly loving or supportive. Farrah had grown accustomed to having a distant relationship with her parents, but her needs changed when her second baby was born. She felt that she wanted her parents to be more involved with her life and her family, and she needed their help. Her long-standing feelings of being abandoned by them really surfaced in the postpartum period. When they were unable to alter their behavior to meet her needs, Farrah felt profoundly disappointed and abandoned, and she began to get depressed.

On a different note, women who have been sexually abused sometimes find labor and delivery to be overwhelming experiences. The intensity, pain, unpredictability, and exposure that are often part of labor and delivery may remind women of the abuse they suffered. Or, if the labor and delivery do not go according to plan, this might elicit feelings of being out of control, similar to the feelings triggered by abuse. These circumstances can trigger PPD.

We will talk later in the book about ways to create and maintain the support you need, and I'll suggest some important ways for letting go and moving on from past hurts so you can get back to enjoying yourself and your time with your new baby.

Body Image Issues

In our thin-obsessed culture, women often find that the weight gain and body changes associated with pregnancy and nursing are downright terrifying. If you feel that being thin defines you and you gain self-worth from maintaining your ideal body, seeing your body change when you are pregnant or after you give birth can be devastating.

Many women feel unattractive when they don't look like a celebrity mom six weeks after pushing out their baby. They feel down on themselves for not "bouncing back" and worry about their attractiveness. If they are not back to their pre-baby weight right away, women often feel that they will be viewed as lazy and overindulgent and they worry that their partner may not be attracted to them. These feelings can be intensely preoccupying and create guilt and distress for new moms. Although these expectations are unrealistic and misguided, many women, unfortunately, have them.

When someone puts excessive pressure on herself to achieve unrealistic physical and weight goals after having a baby, it can be very stressful and another possible trigger for PPD.

Obviously, women who have a history of an eating disorder—such as anorexia nervosa, bulimia nervosa, or binge-eating disorder—are at increased risk of dealing with body image and eating issues in the postpartum period. Women who have a history of an eating disorder often turn to food or focus on their eating habits as a way to gain a sense of control when they are stressed or unhappy. As you know, the postpartum period is a time when women often feel out of control and overwhelmed. Women who are vulnerable to an eating disorder may revert to old habits at this time and this puts them at increased risk of PPD.

Social Risk Factors

This category deals with the risk factors in the world around you, including your home life, social life, and the community and world within which you live.

Stressful Life Events during or after Pregnancy

It is well proven that experiencing a stressful life event can trigger depression. Depressive episodes often follow difficult times in people's lives, such as experiencing the death of a loved one, the end of a relationship, a job loss or unwanted change, a big move, an illness or an accident. If these or other significant stressors affect you immediately prior to pregnancy, during pregnancy, or in the postpartum period, you are at higher risk of developing PPD. Problems with your partner can also increase your risk for having PPD and can also make the recovery process more difficult.

Later in the book I will discuss how you can limit some stressful circumstances and we will talk a lot about how you and your partner can address some of your issues as a couple and learn new skills for working together.

Financial Strain

It is no surprise that women who have significant financial problems during pregnancy or in the postpartum period will feel very stressed and can be at an increased risk for PPD. Related factors, such as unemployment or job loss during pregnancy are also risk factors. (However, it is important to remember that not all women with lower incomes feel stress about money, and vice versa.)

In general, many people worry about money and couples frequently argue about finances. In the early postpartum days when you likely have less money coming in and may have to change how you spend it or how you as a couple share your money, this can be stressful. If there is not enough money to take care of basic needs such as food, medicine, or health care (let alone make life a bit easier with babysitters or house-cleaning help), this will add a significant stress to caring for a newborn.

There are many excellent avenues of support and treatment options that are free or very reasonable, so don't let financial strain hinder your treatment program if you are feeling depressed. I will talk more about this in the chapters to come.

Limited Support

Several scientific studies have shown that women who feel that they do not have meaningful supports during pregnancy and in the postpartum period are at higher risk of having PPD. It is interesting to note that although a woman may appear to have a solid support network, if she does not *feel* that her supports are valuable, then she is in fact at risk of PPD.

Support may come from various sources, including your partner or spouse, other family members, friends and neighbors, colleagues, and other members of your community. Support also comes in different forms. Someone may offer support by bringing meals to your house; someone else may help you by babysitting your child; and another person may be there for you to talk to about your emotions, while others may be able to provide you with helpful baby care ideas or information.

All of the above sources and types of support are valuable and necessary in the postpartum period. Without a system that can provide all or most types of support, a new mother's risk of getting PPD increases. Nobody should navigate the early days of motherhood alone.

For new mothers who have recently moved or immigrated to a new culture where things are done differently, having a new baby can be particularly tough. This is because their important support structures are far less likely to be in place.

In the chapters ahead, there is a lot of useful information about how to create a support network and how to get the kind of help you really need.

Disappointment about the Baby's Gender

Some pregnant women are happy as long as their baby is healthy. For others, the baby's gender is a significant issue. When they find out that they are not having a baby of a certain gender, their deep disappointment (due to personal, family, or cultural reasons) can lead to depression.

In some cultures, male babies are valued more than girls, so mothers may feel like a failure if they have a baby girl who is not prized by their family and larger cultural group. Disappointment about the baby's gender has been shown to be a risk factor for PPD.

Colicky Baby or Sick Newborn

Caring for a newborn baby is a taxing job. It is normal to feel anxious when you are getting to know your baby, learning about his or her cues, and trying to meet your baby's needs. Learning how to soothe your baby can be very difficult and can stir up intense feelings of inadequacy and distress, even at the best of times.

Hopefully you will only have to imagine that when a new mother has a baby who has colic or who cries inconsolably, she is likely to experience significant despair and desperation.

The medical definition of colic is crying more than three hours a day, three days a week for more than three weeks. It is as terrible and difficult as it sounds. Colic often starts a few weeks after birth and can last until a baby is three months old. Unfortunately, there is no clear medical understanding of the causes or treatments for colic, and most parents of colicky babies suffer intensely while trying every possible remedy they can find.

Once you have experienced even a few hours of trying everything you can think of and everything anyone suggests in order to calm your crying baby, it is not hard to imagine how a new mother with a colicky baby develops postpartum depression.

If you are in the unfortunate situation of having a newborn who has been persistently ill, this can also contribute to your risk of PPD. Endless sleepless nights and significant worry are very draining.

The frustration, sense of helplessness, desperation, and exhaustion of trying to calm a chronically fussy baby or cope with a sick newborn can lead to PPD.

Other Child-Related Stressors

Having a baby who is born many weeks prematurely can be very anxiety provoking and stressful. Spending your days in the hospital while your tiny newborn is in an incubator or needs ongoing medical attention is not how you imagined the early days of motherhood to unfold. And if you are sent home from the hospital while your baby must stay there, you may feel cheated of the joy of leaving with your baby in your arms, and feel sad or guilty about being apart from your newborn when you go home to get much-needed rest. The stress and disappointment inherent in this situation can lead to PPD.

If this is not your first child, and your baby is coming home to older siblings, you certainly have your hands full. Taking care of a newborn while trying not to neglect your older kids requires a lot of juggling and much energy. Many women also feel guilty that their older children's lives are disrupted by the arrival of a new baby. You may feel torn in different directions, or feel badly that life as your older children once knew it will no longer be the same and that your attention must now be divided. Later in the book, we will talk about how to deal with your other children when a baby comes home.

Complications with Your Pregnancy or Delivery

While some women are blessed with an easy and uncomplicated pregnancy and delivery, others are not so lucky. Many women develop medical problems during pregnancy and require hospitalization, bed rest, or ongoing medical monitoring. Women who develop obstetrical issues can be at increased risk of having PPD. Research has not yet clarified whether or not the actual medical problem is responsible for increasing the risk of PPD or if it is directly caused by the unexpected and stressful event, or if it is the prolonged hospitalization and isolation associated with these problems.

For women who have unexpected and perhaps traumatic events during delivery, PPD may also develop. We have all heard stories where someone may not have had adequate pain control during labor, or needs an emergency C-section, or the doctors have had to use other emergency delivery methods, such as a vacuum or forceps. Of course, the unpredictability, scariness, and pain of these factors can cause a woman to feel out of control, fearful about her baby's survival, and worried for her own health.

Lena was a physician who had a smooth pregnancy until she was 33 weeks pregnant. When she went to see her obstetrician at that time, she was told she had high blood pressure. The doctor was concerned and asked her to return a few days later to be reassessed. When Lena returned, her blood pressure was still very high, so she had to be admitted to hospital for monitoring. She was forced to stop working, and was assigned to bed rest. This threw Lena for a loop because she had not wrapped things up at work and was worried that she was leaving her own patients in the lurch. While she was in hospital, she began to have premature but strong contractions. Unfortunately, Lena did not get adequate pain control because the epidural was unsuccessful. At the same time, her labor did not progress and the baby's heart rate began to drop. Her obstetrician decided that Lena required an urgent C-section. Because there was difficulty in giving Lena an epidural, she required general anesthetic for the C-section. She was not able to see her baby being born or to hold her daughter right away. Lena described feeling very out of control at the end of her pregnancy when she developed medical problems. Being in the hospital was isolating. She also felt helpless throughout her labor and when her baby was born.

"This is not at all how I planned it," she said when she saw me for depression in the early postpartum period.

Having a less than ideal pregnancy and delivery, and feeling helpless and in pain throughout the experience, can be risk factors for PPD.

Maternal Age

Studies have shown that teenage mothers are more likely to develop PPD, but having children later in life does not seem to contribute to PPD.

This is a good thing, since the average age at which women are having their first child is steadily increasing. There is a significant trend toward women waiting to have babies until later in life, after they have achieved their education goals or established their careers. More and more women are having their first babies when they are in their late thirties and into their forties.

Although being older in itself doesn't predispose women to PPD, sometimes adjustment difficulties arise for women who have had thriving careers and years of disposable income and freedom. It can be shocking to experience the dramatic changes in lifestyle, habits, and independence that accompany motherhood.

Unwanted or Unplanned Pregnancy

Being pregnant when you don't want to be or did not think you could be is both stressful and shocking. Some women who did not plan to get pregnant get excited and embrace the idea after an initial period of shock. Although the timing may not be ideal, and having a baby was not part of "the plan" originally, some women who get pregnant unexpectedly are thrilled to be pregnant and excited to become a mother. But for women who resist or resent being pregnant and dread motherhood throughout their pregnancy, PPD can arise.

Pregnancy after Fertility Treatments
Going through fertility treatments to conceive your child ranks among life's most stressful experiences. If it takes a long time to get pregnant, fertility treatments take a tremendous toll on your physical, emotional, financial, and relationship stability. Financial hardship, marital problems, and emotional and physical pain may linger. If you are unable to address and begin to resolve some of these issues when you are pregnant, they may contribute to PPD.

Breastfeeding Issues

Breastfeeding is a hot topic for new mothers, and especially for those with PPD. Physical, psychological, and social issues are all at play when it comes to nursing. This is really an emotionally charged issue. Although there is no conclusive evidence about the relationship between breastfeeding issues and postpartum depression and anxiety, many women with PPD cite nursing issues as a huge trigger.

Pressure to breastfeed is felt from every angle of a new mother's life. New moms have told me that they feel pressure from hospital staff, family, friends, peers, and partners, all of whom want them to breastfeed exclusively.

If you don't or can't breastfeed for a variety of reasons, you may already feel that you are a failure, or not a good mother, or that you are letting your baby down. The intense pressure to breastfeed triggers larger-than-life feelings of guilt and inadequacy. These negative and self-deprecating thoughts can trigger depressive episodes and severe anxiety. If you don't breastfeed, you may feel that others are passing judgment on your choice and your situation. One mom who decided not to breastfeed told me that she felt she was getting "dirty looks" from the other mothers in her moms' group when she pulled out a bottle to feed her baby, and she is not alone.

Lorie was a 29-year-old first-time mother. She had always thought that she would breastfeed her baby exclusively for six months before introducing a bottle. When she was in the hospital after the birth of her daughter, she tried and tried to get the baby to latch. Regardless of her attempts, she was unable to breastfeed. The hospital staff tried everything to help her succeed at breastfeeding, but nothing seemed to work. Although she realized afterwards that the staff wanted what was best for her, she felt that she was being judged and criticized for not being able to breastfeed. When she went home from the hospital, her struggle to nurse her baby continued. However, she could not make it work and her baby was losing weight. She felt like a failure. Lorie began to get very depressed, and soon developed PPD.

Breastfeeding can be hard! What is supposedly the most natural thing in the world is actually tremendously complicated, and depends on many different things coming together seamlessly at the same time. Latching can be tricky, and your nipples can crack, bleed, and become very painful, and milk spurts out when you least expect it! Although for some new mothers, breastfeeding is straightforward or gets easier with time, this is not always the case. Sometimes babies never learn to latch properly; sometimes moms do not have a sufficient milk supply; or moms cannot nurse because of certain medications they are taking, physical limitations, or because they are returning to work. Also, for women who have been sexually abused in the past, breastfeeding may feel like an invasion of privacy; it can be uncomfortably intimate.

New mothers who tend to be anxious and have perfection-ist personalities often find breastfeeding stressful because they feel uncomfortable not knowing exactly how much milk their child is consuming.

Other new mothers, like Sonia, say that breastfeeding makes them feel "claustrophobic." Sonia felt distressed about nursing because she felt she had to be with her baby at all times and never had time to herself. She could not tolerate the thought that she was the only person who could provide sustenance for the baby. This sense of responsibility and intense obligation triggered feelings of depression and anxiety for Sonia. She opted to breastfeed only part of the time so that others could give the baby a bottle and she could have time for herself.

To add to the complexity of the breastfeeding issue, there has been speculation that women are at risk of developing PPD when they stop breastfeeding. This issue has not been widely studied, but there is some data that is interesting to note. Depres-sion might follow weaning for a few reasons. When a woman stops breastfeeding, her hormones undergo another significant shift. The hormone prolactin remains high when a mother is breastfeeding. Elevated levels of prolactin keep estrogen and progesterone levels relatively low. When a woman stops breast-feeding, prolactin levels drop, and estrogen and progesterone increase. Some researchers have suggested that this additional shift in hormone levels may trigger depression in women who are vulnerable to mood changes when their hormones fluctuate.

And from a psychological perspective, weaning your baby may make you feel down because it may reflect the end of a lovely stage. It may be the last time you breastfeed and it can mean the loss of a sense of intimacy with your baby. For some new mothers, the end of breastfeeding is sad because it is the end of a period of exclusivity. The role that only you could provide for your child can now be fulfilled by other people.

For a host of biological, psychological, and social reasons, breastfeeding issues can contribute to the development of PPD.

Which Risk Factors Can You Control?

Risk Factors You Can Control	Risk Factors beyond Your Control
Depression and anxiety in pregnancy if you are still pregnant	Your personal and family history of mental illness
Thyroid problems	Your history of mood changes due to hormonal fluctuations
Personality traits	Your baby's gender
Negative thinking	Your baby's colic or illness
Your support network	Your age
Body image issues	Pregnancy and delivery complications
Some stressful life events	Some stressful life events
Some financial issues	Some financial issues

There are many controllable risks on this list, and that is a very good thing. It means that you have some power in this situation to limit the chances that you will be affected by PPD. If you do get PPD, you can also limit its impact. Although you may have some risk factors that are beyond your control, don't despair. There may be ways to soften the effect the unchangeable risks have on your current situation, as I will describe in upcoming chapters.

Simply taking charge of your health and well-being in this situation can go a long way. Being proactive and energetically planning for the best possible outcome is very empowering. You should feel proud that you are taking steps to help yourself.

If you already have PPD or if you develop postpartum problems, there is still a lot you can do. Knowing that you have it and knowing what your risks are will really help limit the impact of your PPD on you, your baby, and your family. We will help you to create a plan to address your risks head-on and to get the help you need and the support you deserve.

Risk Factors for PPD, PPA, and PPP

❑ You have depression or anxiety while you are pregnant.

❑ You have a personal and/or family history of mental illness.

❑ You have a history of hormone-related mood problems.

❑ You have a thyroid problem.

❑ You have negative thinking patterns.

❑ You are a worrier or a perfectionist.

❑ You have a history of abuse or significant conflict with your parents.

❑ You have body image issues.

❑ You experience stressful events during pregnancy or when the baby is born.

❑ You have serious money problems.

❑ You have a weak support system.

❑ You are disappointed about your baby's gender.

❑ You have a colicky baby or a sick newborn.

❑ There were complications with your pregnancy or delivery.

❑ You are a teenager.

❑ Your pregnancy was or is unwanted.

❑ You had serious fertility issues.

❑ You have breastfeeding Issues.

Here is what you can do now:

1. Review the list of risk factors.
2. Create your own list of the risks that you can control and change.
3. Stay positive and hopeful regardless of how many or which risk factors you have.
4. Keep reading to see what you need to address and how to do so.

Chapter 3

Do You Have Postpartum Depression?

Now that you know what the risk factors are and which apply to you, let's look at the specific signs and symptoms of PPD.

Unfortunately, there are no definitive blood tests or X-rays that can diagnose postpartum problems. To determine if you have postpartum depression, we look at your signs and symptoms, their severity, how long you have had them, how much they are interfering with your life, and how much they are changing you from your normal self. This chapter will cover the symptoms you may have and some of the things you are experiencing. You will also find out what is normal to experience during the postpartum period and how to distinguish between the symptoms of anxiety and depression and the normal experiences that new moms have. As you know, the myths about PPD already discussed sometimes convince new moms that they are okay when really they are struggling too much. You will learn where to draw this line, and also consider what else might be happening to you if it is not PPD. Finally, this chapter will cover postpartum anxiety problems as well as some rare postpartum emergencies.

Gaining a better grasp of what is "normal" as well as the signs and symptoms of PPD will help you in three essential ways. First, you will be able to clearly understand the causes of the feelings and changes you are going through. Second, if you are suffering from PPD, you can rest assured that you are not alone and you are not going crazy. You will realize that these are symptoms of real, recognized illnesses that have great solutions and proven treatments. And third, you will be able to take all this information to your health care providers to help them understand what you are going through and to set up your treatment plan.

Let's begin by talking about the "normal" range of feelings in the postpartum period. Please don't think that when I use the word "normal" I mean that there are distinct right and wrong ways to react to motherhood. In this case, the word "normal" reflects the range of responses that a mom might have when she has a baby that are expected and common, given the circumstances.

What's Normal?

It is probably an understatement to say that having a baby takes a tremendous toll on a woman's life. Her body, mind, emotions, relationships, and identity undergo a radical transformation. Few other life experiences are as all-encompassing and trans-formative as having a baby. At this time, so many emotions will be swirling around. Hopefully, many of these will be very positive and you will experience intense happiness, deep love and joy.

But even positive and desired situations can also be stressful and stir up less joyful emotions. Many new moms have fears about their new responsibilities and their new role. We all worry about whether or not we will know what to do with a delicate newborn, and most of us are scared about not being able to cope with the demands of motherhood. These are very normal fears. Ambivalence is another common feeling among new moms. Feeling ambivalent means that you have both positive and negative feelings about an experience. You may really love and adore your baby, *but* you also feel overwhelmed and trapped and you miss your old life and your pre-baby sense of freedom and independence. Which new mom has not felt these conflicting feelings? And, of course, there is always guilt. Some moms feel guilty that they have glimmers of doubt about motherhood or occasional frustrations with their baby. Other moms feel guilty if they think that they are not being perfect mothers (whatever that means) or meeting their partners' expectations of them. You may feel guilty about the way you choose to feed your baby, where your baby sleeps, who looks after your baby, about going back to work, or needing to take some time for yourself. All these things are very common and very normal.

Remember, having a baby will rock your world. And even though these feelings are so common, most of your friends will not spontaneously share the more gritty and unpleasant experiences of new motherhood. Moms feel ashamed of upsetting feelings at this supposedly very happy time, but once you start being open about your full range of feelings, you will be amazed about how universal they really are.

So, should you ever worry about having less-than-blissful emotions about motherhood? As long as your unenthusiastic thoughts and feelings come and go, you are okay. Or, if they surface when you are particularly overwhelmed or exhausted, and resolve once you get some respite or rest, there is no need for concern. And there is no need to worry if you are still able to carry on with your life and care for your baby. If you can be honest about your feelings during the less cheery moments of new motherhood, it may be helpful to talk to someone you are close to. If you can open up to your partner, a close friend, or another new mom, you will likely get some understanding and perhaps some good ideas about how to deal with your feelings and cope with your stress. If you feel better after airing your feelings and if they remain in the background while you care for your baby and develop as a mom, then you are okay.

Let's take a look at this chart to see what is "normal" and when to take action:

Symptoms That Are Not Serious	Serious Symptoms
Several days of Baby Blues	Feeling very down or really anxious for more than two weeks
Occasional worries that come and go	Relentless anxiety that never goes away
Negative feelings and thoughts that come and go	Negative feelings that outweigh the positive feelings
You can take care of yourself and your baby	You are unable to cope with your life or your baby
Some escape fantasies	Thoughts about harming yourself or your baby
Poor sleep due to caring for your baby	Not being able to sleep when the baby sleeps at night, or needing to stay in bed all the time
Fatigue	Extreme exhaustion or agitation
Normal appetite with normal fluctuations, i.e., your appetite may increase if you are nursing	Compulsive overeating or ongoing loss of appetite
Some forgetfulness	Severe inability to concentrate and focus
Moments of sadness	Intense feelings of sadness that do not go away
Worries that come and go	Relentless worrying

Needing a break from your responsibilities and from your baby	Avoiding your baby
Wanting to limit visitors and activity	Withdrawing from the world and becoming isolated
Occasional irritability and anger	Feelings of intense anger and irritability

When Baby Brings the Blues

Baby Blues is such a common phenomenon and, fortunately, not one that you need to worry a lot about. Baby Blues is what the vast majority of new moms experience in the early days after they bring their baby home. Fifty to 80 percent of new mothers will at times feel sad, irritable, and occasionally anxious. You may feel you overreact to situations and cry more easily. You may have trouble sleeping and not feel very hungry. Despite feeling "off," women who have Baby Blues can continue to care for their newborn and for themselves. These symptoms usually start around postpartum day three, at the time that your milk comes in. What a coincidence! Baby Blues is brought on by dramatic hormonal changes: estrogen and progesterone levels decrease, and breastfeeding hormones rise. It can also be because exhaustion and the reality that you are a mother are hitting hard.

Baby Blues is more of a common and normal reaction to having a baby and not an illness. The key with Baby Blues is that despite the tears and overwhelming feelings, you enjoy being a mother most of the time and feel happy. It often only lasts a few hours or days and should definitely resolve on its own within two weeks. It is covered here because it is common and you should know what to expect, and if you are at risk of developing PPD, you need to pay close attention to how you are feeling at all times after your baby is born. So if you are at

risk, pay extra attention to whether or not you have Baby Blues
and how intense and long-lasting your symptoms are. If you
have Baby Blues, it is important to let your partner and close
supports know how you are feeling and also educate them
about watching out for any symptoms of PPD, which will be
explained in the pages ahead. Chapters 8 and 9 will discuss in
detail how to involve your partner and other supports in your
postpartum experience and recovery program.

In the meantime, you should know that although Baby
Blues will go away on its own, getting more sleep and recruiting
additional helping hands can go a long way toward easing the
Baby Blues. (In general, these are good postpartum strategies.)
It sounds obvious and everyone tells you to do this, but you
would be amazed by how many women overlook these two
fundamental steps.

Do you have Baby Blues?

❏ I had a baby less than two weeks ago.
❏ I feel very irritable at times.
❏ I have been moody at times.
❏ I cry easily.
❏ I overreact to situations.
❏ I feel a bit anxious at times.
❏ I am still able to care for myself and my baby.
❏ I am mostly enjoying myself and my baby.

If you have checked some or all of these boxes, you may
have Baby Blues. The important thing to do is monitor your

feelings to ensure that they resolve within two weeks and that they do not limit your functioning. After two weeks of continuous Baby Blues, it is time to consider whether or not this is becoming something more serious. Please do not wait months before taking action and talking to your doctor. This is precious time that you need not waste.

The Big "D" Word: Postpartum Depression

Now, let's talk about PPD. PPD looks and feels a lot like regular depression, but it happens to 15–20 percent of new moms after the baby is born. Symptoms can begin at anytime within the first year after delivery, but the highest risk period is within the first month after birth.

Abby was a 31-year-old married woman who came to see me because she began feeling distressed during the delivery of her first daughter. She had always wanted to have a vaginal birth, with no epidural. Unfortunately, during labor, the baby developed some medical complications and an emergency C-section was necessary. With this unexpected turn of events, and the loss of her dreams of having a nonmedical and "natural" labor and delivery, Abby began to feel very out of control. This feeling only escalated when she went home with her newborn, and she then developed feelings of depression.

Jennifer, on the other hand, sailed through labor and had an easy delivery. Her mood, however, slowly declined over the first few weeks and months of her baby's life. She felt overwhelmed by her lack of sleep, new role as a mother, and isolation. She felt as if she was out of sync with the rest of the world and she missed the predictability of her work and the sense of accomplishment she derived from her professional life. It was not until Jennifer's son, Jack, was about three months old that she developed a full-blown depression.

You may be surprised to learn that for about 25 percent of women with PPD, depressive symptoms actually began during pregnancy and were never treated or addressed, so they got worse after the baby was born. If you are reading this while you are pregnant and suspect that you might be depressed, act now! Read on to learn how.

> **PPD may begin:**
> - during pregnancy
> - in the first month postpartum
> - during the first year of your baby's life

Especially if you know you are at risk, monitor yourself closely for the first few months after the baby is born. You will learn which signs to watch for. This does not mean that you should be scared or worried, but be aware of the signs and symptoms and let your family and your supports know about them too. By knowing the signs and symptoms and sharing this information, you can act quickly if they develop and nip PPD in the bud.

Most women are scared that an exaggerated form of PPD will arrive all at once—that you go to bed feeling normal one night and wake up homicidal the next day. That *would* be terrifying. Luckily, that isn't at all the case: PPD will not, unlike what many people think, manifest as "crazy" behavior that begins as soon as the baby pops out. In reality, PPD usually begins slowly, and women are fully aware that they are not feeling quite right.

Here are the fears I most often hear: "I'll suddenly lose my mind and find myself standing over the baby with a butcher knife." Or, "I will suddenly wake up to find myself, babe in arms, standing on a busy street, about to jump in front of a bus." These fears are directly linked to sensationalized news stories rather than the hundreds of thousands of common PPD stories. The major concern is that this illness starts suddenly, takes over your mind, and makes you do "crazy" and dangerous things. However, these stories are examples of untreated postpartum psychosis, not cases of the much more common PPD. By learning the symptoms of PPD, you will know what PPD *really* looks like and you will be able to stop it swiftly.

Recognizing PPD: What to Watch out for

Let's start by understanding in detail what PPD feels like. Depression is an illness that makes you feel deeply distraught and intensely sad. It usually prevents you from taking joy from your life. But it also affects how your body functions and can hinder your ability to think clearly. The symptoms of PPD fall into three main areas: (1) physical symptoms; (2) symptoms that impact your thinking (cognitive symptoms); and (3) emotional symptoms. Before being officially diagnosed with PPD, your symptoms would have to persist for two weeks. However, there is no reason to wait two weeks before taking action. Below is a list of signs that you, your partner, your family and friends can watch out for. (At the back of the book, there is a copy of the Edinburgh Postnatal Depression Scale, a commonly used screening tool, which you can also look at to see if you have PPD.) As you read this chapter, jot down the symptoms that apply to you. Later in the book, there will be many helpful solutions you can implement on your own and great information about getting the help you need.

Physical Symptoms
These symptoms of PPD affect your body and how it works.

"I Just Can't Sleep"
Ahhh sleep! Sleep is an elusive dream for almost every new mother, so how do we know if not getting enough sleep is "normal" or part of a larger problem? Most new moms desperately want more sleep and scheme about how to get it when

and where they can. Of course, given the opportunity, usually a new mom is out like a light the moment the baby's tucked in. However, if you are unable to sleep at night on an ongoing basis, even when your baby is sleeping, it is cause for concern. If you feel totally exhausted and want to sleep, but cannot calm yourself down enough to fall asleep, or if you lie in bed while worries and doubts race through your mind, this is a problem. Poor sleep is a very sensitive indicator of postpartum mental health problems. The inability to sleep, or insomnia, is one of the most common symptoms of PPD.

Sometimes women with PPD have the opposite of insomnia, and find that they need and want to sleep all the time. They cannot care for their baby because they are always asleep. For these new mothers, sleeping may be the way they withdraw from their newborn and try to forget about their new role.

Being tired is simply a reality of new motherhood, but insomnia or a constant and incapacitating need to sleep is a key indicator of PPD.

Changes in Energy

It is very normal for a new mother to feel exhausted. After being unable to sleep at the end of pregnancy, enduring a long and painful labor and delivery or having a C-section, and caring for a newborn 24/7, fatigue is an expected part of the package.

As with difficulty sleeping, there are indicators that help us to distinguish between reasonable fluctuations in energy and symptoms of PPD. These have to do with intensity and duration. If you feel incapacitated by exhaustion and cannot function to take care of yourself or your baby for several days on end, this is a symptom of PPD.

While some women with PPD feel slowed down, others feel too "revved up." Some say that even though they feel exhausted, they are unable to sit still and they feel jittery. Jamie described feeling that she had an "internal motor that didn't turn off," which left her feeling very agitated. Pay attention to your energy level. If it feels extreme in either direction, this could be a symptom of PPD. It may also mean that you have an underlying medical problem, such as a thyroid disorder or anemia.

Changes in Appetite, Weight Loss, or Weight Gain

Most people who have depression find that their appetite is affected by the illness. Some people simply cannot eat and they lose weight when they get depressed, while others overeat and gain weight.

Among women who get PPD, some feel compelled to overeat and find that food is their sole source of comfort. Other mothers lose their appetites, are turned off by food, and have to force themselves to eat.

Think about what has happened to your appetite. If it has radically changed, this is another important marker for PPD and something to discuss with your doctor.

Cognitive Symptoms

These symptoms of PPD impact how your brain works.

Difficulty Concentrating or Poor Decision Making

New mothers know that "baby brain" really exists. New moms often complain about being forgetful and disorganized in the days and months after they give birth. It seems that the combination of sleep deprivation, stress, and fluctuating hormones deprives the brain of the ability to function at full capacity. In normal depression, the brain's capacity to think, make decisions, and concentrate is compromised. This is compounded in postpartum depression.

For moms with PPD, "baby brain" goes one step further: You may find that you have trouble concentrating on mindless reality-TV shows or that you forget what you are saying in mid-conversation. Or you may have tremendous trouble making even the most inconsequential decision.

Bella could not think clearly or make any decisions without agonizing. She changed her baby's outfit seven times before leaving the house because she was so worried she would choose an outfit that was inappropriate for the weather. She was riddled with self-doubt and could not focus on thinking through the situation in order to make a decision.

Don't worry if you forget your sunhat or can't find your shopping list. But if your forgetfulness becomes scary, or you find it unusually distressing to make the smallest choices, then these could be symptoms of PPD.

Emotional Symptoms
The following symptoms of PPD affect your feelings.

From the Bottom of the Black Hole: Depressed Mood
Brooke Shields suffered from PPD and described feeling "like my life was over and I would never be happy again." Everyone describes the experience of depression a little differently. It ranges from an ongoing sense of "being really sad" or "not at all like myself," to feeling "nothing" to feeling "intense misery."

Depression is not just feeling down for a few hours or a few days. It is intense sadness that lasts for several days on end. If you are depressed, you are unlikely to enjoy your daily life or to laugh like you normally do. You probably also feel plagued by very negative and dark thoughts about yourself, the world around you, and your future. Depression makes you feel hopeless, as though things will never improve, and you cannot imagine feeling better.

"I Can't Stop Worrying"

We've all experienced anxiety at some point. Medically, we define anxiety as intense worry that is more than expected for a given circumstance, but how does one apply that in real life? What is "more than expected"? Anxiety is very often a major part of what women with PPD struggle with, and an important cue in diagnosis. Practically every mom will have a night of lying awake with worry—this is a huge life change. Of course, as we already discussed, you will think about what this baby means to your future, about your new responsibilities, and you will occasionally feel totally overwhelmed, imagining the worst scenarios. A sleepless night of worry is not in itself a symptom of PPD. Anxiety becomes problematic when it is relentless and uncontrollable. This type of anxiety is a symptom of PPD or other anxiety disorders, which will be described later.

Jill was a 28-year-old new mother who came to see me after the birth of her third son. She was exhausted and depressed. She was unwilling to sleep at night or whenever her baby was asleep because she was terrified that her baby would suddenly stop breathing in his crib. Jill's anxiety prompted her to sit by her son at all times and to hold a mirror up to his face whenever she could not detect movement or an obvious sign that he was alive. If she could see the baby's breath condensing on the mirror, she felt reassured for only a few minutes.

Tabitha was also a very anxious new mother. She worried constantly that her baby girl was developing one illness or another. If the baby coughed, Tabitha worried that she might have pneumonia; if she spit up, Tabitha thought she might have celiac disease. She made daily phone calls to her pediatrician and visited the pediatrician's office weekly for checkups. After visiting her baby's doctor, she would be reassured briefly—until she found a new symptom to worry about.

Problematic anxiety is often accompanied by physical symptoms. Tightness in the throat or a gripping feeling in the chest, dizziness, or a knot in the stomach are some of the things that people with very bad anxiety may experience, in addition to the gnawing feelings of constant worry and spinning doubts and fears. When someone has an anxious thought, adrenaline kicks in and triggers physical symptoms (racing heart, shortness of breath, shaking, blurred vision, etc.) and then the person interprets these to mean that she is going to die or is going "crazy." Of course, this makes the anxious feelings worse, and then she is caught in a vicious anxiety cycle.

When new moms like Jill or Tabitha spend significantly more of their time fretting, doubting, and worrying than enjoying and living, anxiety becomes problematic. When thoughts and activities are consumed and guided by anxiety, or the physical feelings of anxiety do not go away, they are hallmarks of PPD or postpartum anxiety disorder.

> Anxiety is very common with PPD.

"Nothing Makes Me Happy"
If you have PPD, it can be hard to take pleasure in anything at all. Nothing in life gives you joy and this is a distinct change from your normal experience of the world. Time with your family and friends, fun activities, sex, and everything else can feel dull.

"Help! I Feel Nothing for My Baby"
Having a baby is *supposed* to be one of the most joyous times of your life. We expect it to be a time filled with happiness. Although nobody will tell you that motherhood is always

idyllic, most moms experience a great deal of pleasure from their children much of the time. One of the most painful aspects of PPD is that it becomes difficult, if not impossible, to enjoy your baby.

Carrie was a 32-year-old primary schoolteacher who had a magic touch with children and loved being around kids. She dreamed about the day she could have a baby of her own, and she and her partner decided to try to have a baby as soon as possible after they got married. Fortunately, Carrie got pregnant right away and really enjoyed her pregnancy. Soon after her son was born, she developed PPD. When she was depressed, Carrie felt she could not connect with her baby boy and that she did not love him. She dreaded being alone with her son and counted the minutes until her husband returned home from work so she could hand the baby over to him and be by herself. Others would comment on her adorable baby and what a "natural" mother she must be, given that she was a wonderful and experienced teacher, but she just could not feel love and affection for her son. Carrie worried that she was a horrible mother because she did not enjoy being with the baby she had wanted for so long, and she felt ashamed of these feelings.

Although having a baby is challenging and it is completely normal for a mother to need a break from her child and to want time for herself, when a new mom has trouble enjoying her baby most of the time, this is often a significant marker of PPD.

Some people fall in love immediately with their newborn, while it takes others longer to develop a deep love for their baby. For many women, the bond with their baby deepens with time. Don't worry if you are not overcome instantly with intense love for your child. As long as your love grows and you are making an effort to connect with your baby and to deepen the bond, everything is fine. But if you find that you are avoiding your child, do not want to care for the baby, or have no feelings at all or feelings of resentment or intense rejection, this is often a sign of PPD. By getting appropriate help to address these feelings and your PPD, you can strengthen your bond with your baby.

"I Feel So Guilty"

Allison came into my office with her three-month-old baby and said, "If having a baby is supposed to be the happiest event of my life and if women are supposed to naturally want to be mothers and to instantly fall in love with their newborn babies, there is something really wrong with me. I sure don't feel the way I'm supposed to feel, and I feel terrible about that."

Most women with PPD do not feel the way that they think new mothers are "supposed" to feel. Because their reactions to their babies and to motherhood are often incongruous with what they think they *should* feel, and also with how they think other new moms feel, guilt looms large. They may believe, like Allison, that they are flawed, or that they never should have had a baby. Of course, there are as many reactions to being a mother as there are mothers. But new mothers who are depressed frequently tend to think that all other mothers love their new role and are thriving, while they are horrible people who cannot make it work.

There are countless cultural and social messages about what it takes to be the perfect mother and about the "right way" to raise your child. In our culture, where the "breast is best" notion is widespread, many women feel guilty if they do not breastfeed. Other women feel guilty because they worry they are not stimulating their child sufficiently if they do not enroll their baby in music, sign language, and baby yoga.

Unfortunately, guilt and motherhood often go hand in hand. Every mom you know would probably admit to feeling guilty at some point each day. As mothers, we are all situated somewhere along the guilt continuum at any given moment and our position on this continuum changes every day with new situations. There is no particular point at which you definitively have PPD, but prolonged, intense guilt that makes you doubt yourself and feel badly about who you are is a very strong indicator of PPD and something you need to monitor closely.

It is all too easy to intensify feelings of guilt or shame by feeling guilty and shameful about having these emotions. Try to be kind to yourself and realistic about how common your experiences are. There are ways to tune into these negative thought patterns and guide them toward a positive track; I'll talk in detail about that in Chapter 4.

"Get Me away from These People!"

When I asked Julie if she was withdrawing from the people in her life, she said, "I hate everyone, especially my husband." Yikes! But she actually summed up how many women with PPD feel toward others. It is common for moms with PPD to feel intensely irritable and easily enraged. Of course, if you feel constant rage, you want to isolate yourself from the rest of the world.

Also, women with PPD are often ashamed and embarrassed that they have this illness. As a result, they feel out of step with other new mothers they meet who seem to be adjusting well, and they want to avoid acquaintances for fear of being seen as a defective mother and a disappointment. These feelings contribute to further isolation because depressed moms feel they don't belong in any new moms' groups or activities and they avoid people they already know.

Don't worry if you occasionally bark or snap at your partner (But don't tell them I said that.), or if you want to limit visitors.

But if your anger feels overwhelming and constant and you always avoid going out, this can be a symptom of PPD. As you find out how you can feel better, these feelings will diminish.

"The Only Way Is Out": Escape Fantasies

Many new moms have "escape fantasies" at particularly rough moments in the day. They may have fleeting thoughts about walking out the front door of their house to flee from their life, their overwhelming new responsibility, and all that it entails. These types of thoughts are not uncommon among new mothers and are nothing to worry about if they happen rarely and quickly subside after a few minutes of calm. After all, caring for a newborn can be really rough, and it is normal to want respite in a tough situation. This is your mind's way of telling you that you need a break and are feeling overwhelmed.

Escape fantasies are not a symptom of PPD if they are few and far between. But if you find that you cannot stop thinking about getting away, that you don't want to care for your baby at all, or that your baby and your family would be better off without you, this is different. This signals an underlying postpartum emotional problem.

Scary Thoughts

It is not uncommon for women with postpartum depression to have intrusive thoughts about harming their baby.

Deana's "scary thoughts" began soon after she brought her son home from the hospital. When she was preparing dinner in the kitchen with a large knife, she suddenly felt that she might turn the knife on her baby and injure him. She could not get this gruesome image out of her mind. As the days progressed, she continued to have thoughts that she would harm her son with the knife. She began to avoid going into the kitchen, to avoid using any knife, and she was unable to be alone with her son because she was afraid she might hurt him.

The key thing with these unwanted and terrifying thoughts is that they are *just* thoughts. They are not actions. Having these thoughts does not mean you are acting on them. It is totally understandable that you are afraid of having these thoughts and hate having them. If they occur once in a while and become less frequent and less intense, don't worry. But if you cannot get the scary thoughts out of your mind and they surface all the time, and you find yourself avoiding people or places or things as a result, this is a symptom of concern. Again, it does not mean that you are going to *do* anything, but this is likely a symptom of PPD or of postpartum obsessive-compulsive disorder, which we will talk about shortly. Regardless of your exact diagnosis, the important thing to remember is that these are simply thoughts, you are not going "crazy," and you still have a firm grasp on reality. Being scared of the thoughts is a good thing. Your fear means that you are aware of the difference between right and wrong. You will not act on these thoughts.

> Even if your feelings and thoughts seem overwhelming, you are not going crazy, and you will get through this.

There are more serious symptoms of PPD that are considered an emergency, including suicidal and homicidal thoughts. Postpartum mania and psychosis are also crises that can arise in the postpartum period and need immediate attention. These urgent problems are discussed at the end of the chapter along with suggestions about what to do if they are happening to you.

Do you have PPD?

❏ My mood is very depressed most of the time.

❏ I am not enjoying anything.

❏ I do not want to care for my baby.

❏ I am having trouble bonding with my baby.

❏ My sleep is off: I have trouble sleeping even when my baby sleeps, or I sleep too much.

❏ My energy level is off: My energy is too low or I feel agitated.

❏ My appetite is off: I have no appetite or I am overeating.

❏ I cannot focus.

❏ I have trouble making decisions.

❏ My memory is terrible.

❏ I feel very nervous.

❏ I feel very guilty.

❏ I am very irritable and angry.

❏ I do not want to be around other people.

❏ I am crying a lot.

❏ I feel hopeless about the future.

❏ I am experiencing scary thoughts that do not go away.

❏ I have frequent thoughts about leaving or ending my life.

The Degrees of PPD:

PPD is not the same for every woman. Some women may have mild cases while others are more severely affected. Each of these is a real illness that needs attention. Here is what the different degrees of PPD look like:

Mild: You do not fully enjoy being a mom or much else in your life these days and you have some symptoms of depression, but you can still go through the motions to do what you need to do to take care of yourself and your baby. There is room for improvement, but you are getting by.

Moderate: You feel down all the time and have trouble being a mom and connecting with your baby. You have symptoms of depression and are not at all your normal self. It is really hard to get through each day.

Severe: Your mood is extremely depressed and you have most of the symptoms of depression. You are unable to look after your own needs and you just cannot attend to your baby.

In addition to the Baby Blues and PPD, there are a few other common postpartum conditions that you should also know about in more detail. These are postpartum anxiety disorders (PPA).

Postpartum Anxiety Disorders

Although postpartum anxiety disorders have been studied less than PPD, they are also common problems. Some researchers even believe they are more common than postpartum depression. Regardless of the numbers, there is no doubt that having a postpartum anxiety disorder takes a significant toll on the woman who is suffering. In this category there are four main illnesses: (1) generalized anxiety disorder; (2) panic disorder;

(3) obsessive-compulsive disorder; and (4) posttraumatic stress disorder.

Anxiety disorders are common in the postpartum period. Sometimes they happen alone, and at other times, women with PPA also develop PPD. Debilitating and isolating panic attacks that continue for weeks on end may make someone feel very depressed, or the scary thoughts of obsessive-compulsive disorder can lead to PPD. At the same time, many women with PPD endure significant anxiety symptoms. I described some of these earlier: excessive worrying, agitation, and intrusive thoughts. But for women with PPD, their major symptom is feeling depressed.

Feel confused? You will see that there is some overlap of symptoms between the postpartum anxiety disorders and PPD. Sometimes the dividing line between the different diagnoses is not crystal clear, but ultimately your final diagnosis is not the most important thing. The most important thing is that you recognize that you are suffering, understand as best you can your symptoms and their causes, and realize that you are not alone. After recognizing your problem, you can find the support and treatment you need.

The myths that were described in Chapter 1 often also keep women with anxiety disorders from getting medical care. The myth that it is normal to feel badly and nervous after you have had a baby can prevent women from realizing that their anxiety is problematic. While every new mother occasionally worries about some things, this worry should not be debilitating.

The causes of PPA and PPD are similar, as are the risk factors. If you have a personal or family history of anxiety problems or have always been a big worrier, the hormonal changes of pregnancy and the postpartum period and the stress of caring for a newborn can trigger a postpartum anxiety disorder. But again, stay hopeful, because there is so much you can do to limit PPA. Also, the treatments for PPA are effective and safe, just as they are for PPD.

Still, you should know specifically what the anxiety disorders feel like so you can determine if this is what you are experiencing. Then you, or you and your partner, can use your understanding to create your own care plan, and you can approach your health care provider armed with knowledge. This way, he or she can help to customize an ideal recovery and treatment plan for you. There will be detailed information about what you can do to help yourself and how to get your doctor to help you succeed. But before discussing getting help, let's examine the postpartum anxiety disorders in more detail.

Generalized Anxiety Disorder (GAD)

New moms who have GAD worry excessively about pretty much everything. They worry that they may be feeding their baby too little; that their baby is sleeping too much; that their baby is not meeting his or her milestones; and that the littlest sniffle may turn into pneumonia.

This is different from the "normal" worries of all new mothers because moms with GAD cannot be reassured and cannot turn off their worry, despite knowing that they are worrying too much. Also, their worries consume a large portion of each day and night and compromise their ability to function and care for themselves and their baby. About 4–8 percent of new moms are affected by GAD.

In addition to the never-ending stream of worries and feeling on edge, new moms with GAD might also experience physical symptoms, such as headaches, muscle tension in their necks and shoulders, knots in their stomachs, difficulty sleeping, or diarrhea.

Do you have generalized anxiety disorder?

❏ I worry way too much about too many things.

❏ I cannot control my anxiety.

❏ When I'm anxious, I also:

- – feel jittery
- – feel exhausted
- – cannot focus
- – feel irritable
- – have muscle tension
- – cannot sleep well

Panic Disorder

If you have ever had a panic attack, then you know how horrible the sudden and unexpected intense fear—coupled with overwhelming physical sensations, such as a pounding heart, difficulty breathing, dizziness, vision changes, numbness, tingling, and sweating—can be. It is no wonder that people who are having panic attacks feel that they are "going crazy" or are "going to die" during the attacks, which may last for about 10 minutes.

One sunny day, Victoria, a self-described shopaholic, went to a mall with her adorable three-month-old daughter. Suddenly, she felt really nervous, got dizzy, felt that her head was pounding, and sensed tingling in both arms. She "freaked out," thought she was having a stroke, and left the mall immediately. When Victoria got home, she told her partner what had happened. Over the next few days, whenever she left the house, Victoria felt nervous and some of the same symptoms returned, so she would head straight home. Soon she was scared to go out because she worried that she would pass out in public and that she would look "ridiculous" and nobody would be able to help her. When Victoria began to dread being alone with her baby because she feared she would not be able to care for her if she was debilitated by a panic attack, she knew she had to get some help.

Sometimes panic attacks are triggered by specific situations, but more often than not, there are no identifiable triggers and they happen out of the blue. This can be really scary and leaves those who have had one panic attack to worry about having another one. Often the worry about having another panic attack becomes more debilitating than the panic attacks themselves.

Panic attacks affect about 1-2 percent of pregnant women and new moms. Please know that you are not going crazy and that you are not going to die if you have episodes similar to Victoria's. You are having panic attacks. The best way to deal with panic attacks is to get help when they begin, so that they do not negatively impact you or your baby. You will learn how to get appropriate care in the pages ahead.

Do you have panic disorder?

❑ I have had a panic attack (pounding heart, shortness of breath, sweating, shaking, choking, chest pain, upset stomach, dizziness).

❑ I worry about losing control or going crazy when I have a panic attack.

❑ I dread having another panic attack.

❑ I worry about being unable to care for my baby if I have a panic attack.

❑ I avoid going to certain places or doing certain things out of fear of having a panic attack again.

Obsessive-Compulsive Disorder (OCD)

The previous section covered scary thoughts that new moms may have. These may be symptoms of PPD if they come and go as part of your depression. But if the thoughts take on a life of their own and are persistent, extremely upsetting, and you cannot get rid of them no matter how hard you try, they are called "obsessions."

You might have OCD if you are suffering from obsessions or if you have compulsions, which are repetitive behaviors or rituals that you may do to make the obsessions go away or to feel less anxious about them. But these compulsions can often become problematic on their own. For example, if you are afraid of being contaminated by germs, you may develop washing rituals that take up hours of your day and interfere with you getting things done.

The thoughts and behaviors associated with OCD become pathological when they are very upsetting, or if they take up too much time and get in the way of your day-to-day life and functioning.

Two to 3 percent of new moms have OCD. They often have obsessions about harming their baby, either on purpose or by mistake.

One week after coming home from the hospital, Kiley suddenly started to have scary thoughts that she might hit her baby's head against their glass coffee table. Every time Kiley saw the coffee table, she had to leave the living room. Soon she was unable to enter the living room at all, and after a few weeks she would not go downstairs in her home. She then asked her husband to get rid of the coffee table. Kiley also became frightened of being alone with her son for fear that she might harm him. She knew these thoughts were wrong and did not want to act on them, but felt like a "monster" for having these consuming thoughts.

Other women develop obsessions about their babies being contaminated. They may then develop cleaning compulsions and spend countless hours scrubbing themselves or their homes to ensure cleanliness. There are also checking, counting, and ordering compulsions. Other new moms have intrusive thoughts about drowning their babies during bath time or smothering them with a blanket. These are truly scary and are the height of frightening experiences for those who have them. Women with OCD feel terribly guilty, ashamed, and distressed about their symptoms. Once again, those myths about PPD and PPA can really be damaging because women with OCD feel terrible about what they are going through and often keep silent. They try to ignore them, hoping the bad thoughts will go away. Of course, you cannot *just stop* the thoughts or the acts when you have OCD, even though you desperately want to.

Please be reassured that *there has never been a documented case of a new mom with OCD harming her child.* OCD is a very distressing illness because it makes you think and feel things that you never imagined you could think or feel, and you cannot understand why these strange thoughts are clouding your mind. All you want to do is love and care for your baby and you feel like your mind is sabotaging you. The key is that these are only thoughts—you are not a monster, and you can get excellent help to feel better and put your worried mind at ease. Treatment will be discussed soon.

Do you have obsessive compulsive disorder?

❑ I have repeated intrusive and inappropriate thoughts that make me very anxious.

❑ I realize my mind is playing tricks on me.

❑ I try to ignore these thoughts, but they won't go away.

❑ I have repetitive behaviors or rituals.

❑ My obsessions or compulsions take up more than one hour of the day and interfere with my life.

Posttraumatic Stress Disorder (PTSD)

When labor and delivery go drastically wrong, and a woman feels stripped of power and control, she can develop PTSD. Having an emergency C-section, a dramatic delivery, or feeling overwhelming pain or lack of support can trigger PTSD. Some women who had earlier experiences of abuse or assault may also get PTSD after labor and delivery because they are reminded of previous emotional and physical pain and of feeling out of control.

The main symptoms of PTSD are having nightmares or flashbacks of a traumatic event. New moms with PTSD also feel on edge much of the time. They may try to numb their feelings by getting drunk or high on drugs, and they avoid triggers that remind them of the traumatic event. Sometimes that means they avoid being with their babies because the babies remind them of the hard time they had.

The symptoms of PTSD and the underlying issues need to be addressed and will respond well to talk therapy and medication, as will be discussed.

Do you have posttraumatic stress disorder?

❏ I experienced a traumatic event.
❏ I have had many disturbing memories, nightmares, or flashbacks about the event.
❏ I feel numb.
❏ I avoid people, places, or events that remind me of the trauma, including my baby.
❏ I feel consistently edgy.

Postpartum Mental Health Emergencies

Although 99 percent of new moms will never have suicidal or homicidal thoughts, a manic episode, or become psychotic, here is some information about these emergencies just in case. At the end of the chapter is a list of urgent symptoms that need immediate attention, as well as what to do if these problems arise. If you have had any of these troubles in the past or if you are at high risk for them, please read this section and share it with your family and your physician, so that you can be prepared and take action, if necessary.

Suicidal Thoughts

When suicidal thoughts arise, it is usually after a new mom has been suffering with depression or anxiety for some time, alone and in silence. The thoughts often emerge when women think that they are terrible mothers, that they should never have had a child, and that they are "bad" for feeling as they do. The PPD myths that treatments are unavailable and that women should feel ashamed of themselves only compound this, which is why they are addressed in this book.

Sometimes suicidal thoughts might occur when you are feeling particularly overwhelmed or frustrated. At those times, you may feel that ending your life is your only way to cope. At other times, you may feel desperately depressed and constantly think about and plan how to take your life. Both of these are serious situations that indicate you have PPD. If you are having thoughts about ending your life and you have a plan, this is an emergency. Please read the emergency section at the end of this chapter. My hope is that armed with the information in this book, you will not reach this stage of depression.

Homicidal Ideation

Fixating on and planning to harm other people, particularly your baby, is a symptom of serious PPD and, more likely, of postpartum psychosis. Unlike a person experiencing scary thoughts, someone with homicidal ideation does not feel anxiety. This is a rare symptom and one that develops after someone has had long-standing and severe, untreated PPD or psychosis. This is not a symptom that occurs in isolation or without warning. Again, if you have these thoughts, this is an emergency, so please turn to the end of the chapter to learn what to do now.

Mania

Postpartum mania is also known as the Baby Pinks, which at first can look like the opposite of depression or "the blues." When someone is manic, her mood can be euphoric and she may seem like the life of the party. She may be on energy over-drive even after getting only minimal sleep for days on end. She may speak very quickly, enthusiastically, and loudly about various ideas and plans. She may not complete one thought before excitedly jumping to the next one. She may describe her thoughts as "racing."

To a drained and sluggish new mom, the Baby Pinks can sound like an enviable condition. However, the reality is that the initial euphoria and excitement that a manic mother might have turns into intense irritability and extreme moodiness. And as the insomnia continues, her energy usually becomes destructive and chaotic. She may seem to be getting a lot of things done, but she is really a whirling dervish who is so disorganized that she cannot complete anything. It is as if she spirals out of control and cannot slow down her speech or her actions. She may also do impulsive things, like spend money she does not have or become sexually promiscuous. If the manic episode continues, a woman might also lose touch with reality and may develop ideas about having "special powers" or grandiose notions about what she can and cannot do. This could put a woman at risk of endangering herself or her child. We will talk more about psychosis in a minute.

Women who have a personal history or a strong family history of bipolar disorder have the highest risk of having a postpartum manic episode because of hormonal changes after birth as well as the intense sleep deprivation that accompanies this stage. However, even new moms who have had bipolar disorder or a manic episode in the past are not destined to become manic. In fact, they are more likely to have depression after their baby is born than to become manic, or they may experience a combination of symptoms of both depression and mania. It is rare that someone who has no history of bipolar disorder develops postpartum mania. Mania is a treatable problem. It usually requires medication, as will be discussed. The key is to act swiftly at the first signs of the problem to prevent it from getting out of hand.

Postpartum Psychosis (PPP)

Postpartum psychosis is what every woman I see in my office fears most, but let me reassure you: PPP is an extremely rare condition that occurs in one or two out of every 1,000 new mothers. You have a greater chance of winning your local lottery than of having this problem. PPP in itself is not a specific illness, but a very severe form of an underlying bipolar disorder, psychotic depression or another psychotic illness. Remember, you are most at risk of having postpartum psychosis if you have had it before, if you have a history of serious bipolar disorder, psychotic depression or a psychotic illness such as schizophrenia, or a close family member has had postpartum psychosis or schizophrenia or bipolar disorder. If you do develop postpartum psychosis but act quickly, it is treatable and you can make an excellent recovery.

Now that I have allayed some of your concerns about PPP, you should educate your partner and close support system about it. The quicker you recognize it and take action, the better the outcome for you and for your family.

Postpartum psychosis usually begins within the first five days of the postpartum period. A new mom with postpartum psychosis appears dramatically different from her normal self. She may seem confused and disorganized and in her own world. Her behavior appears very strange. She may seem agitated and roam aimlessly and may not sleep at all.

Someone is psychotic when she has lost touch with reality, which means that she is having experiences and thoughts that she perceives as real, even though they are only in her head. For example, she may hear voices that only she can hear, but she thinks they actually exist. These are called auditory hallucinations. She might also have visual hallucinations and see things that are not really there. And her thinking may be delusional. This means that she has firmly held beliefs that something is really happening when it isn't. Delusions might be in the form of paranoid fears that someone is trying to harm her or her child. And some psychotic women have grandiose delusions about having special powers, such as the ability to walk on water or to heal all the illness in the world. Take Gisele, for example.

Gisele was a 32-year-old lawyer who suffered from bipolar disorder. She had a few depressive episodes and was hospitalized for a psychotic manic episode at age 23. She had been doing well since that time and was stabilized on medication. However, she stopped her medication while she was pregnant. Gisele began to behave strangely three days after her baby was born. She was still in the obstetrics ward when she began to think that whenever she heard an ambulance siren, "the officials" were coming to get her and were trying to take her new baby away from her.

She became very suspicious of the hospital staff and thought they were talking about what an awful mother she was. She then acknowledged that she was hearing voices telling her to flee from the hospital with her newborn so that the baby would not be taken away from her. When the hospital staff learned about Gisele's psychotic paranoid thoughts and her auditory hallucinations, she was seen by a psychiatrist. Because she needed to be monitored, she was transferred to the psychiatric ward at the hospital. Gisele responded well to medication and her paranoid thoughts stopped. Once that happened, she was able to return home with her family and became an excellent mother to her baby.

Psychotic symptoms need urgent medical attention because women truly believe they are experiencing these things and may act on their thoughts and ideas. For example, a psychotic new mom who hears voices commanding her to harm her baby may act on these thoughts. Women who are psychotic cannot distinguish between what is real or imaginary and they are unlikely to think they have a problem or to get help. In contrast, when women who have PPD, PPA, or OCD have thoughts about harming their baby, they know that what they are thinking is wrong and are scared of their thoughts and experiences.

And that is why your partner, family, and friends need to understand this illness if you are at risk. If they act quickly to contact your doctor, you can be treated and recover fully. Women with PPP often need to be hospitalized to ensure a full and speedy recovery. Treatment often consists of medication at first, such as antipsychotic medication and sleeping pills, and can be followed by talk therapy too, once someone is feeling better and not experiencing psychotic symptoms.

Please consider four things about PPP:

1. PPP is very rare.

2. PPP almost always happens to women with a history of severe mental illness. If you are at risk, meet with your doctor or psychiatrist and develop a postpartum care plan.

3. Let your partner and family know if you are at risk so they can help you plan in advance and they can recognize the signs and get help for you immediately, if necessary.

4. Treatments work well and you will recover.

Postpartum Emergencies

1. You have thoughts about killing yourself and you have a plan.
2. You have homicidal ideations
3. You have not been able to sleep or eat for over two days.
4. You are unable or unwilling to care for yourself or your baby.
5. You are hearing voices telling you to do something.
6. You are seeing things that are not there.
7. You have paranoid delusions that someone is trying to harm you or your baby.
8. You feel you have lost touch with reality.
9. You feel agitated constantly.
10. You are definitely not yourself.

ACT NOW:

1. *Tell your partner or family or friends:* Telling other people what you are going through will ensure that they can help you get the help you need immediately.

2. *Call your health care provider:* If you are being treated by a physician or a therapist, you need to inform him or her immediately. He or she should take this situation very seriously and assess you immediately. If your health care provider is unable to do so, you should be referred to a psychiatrist urgently or should go to your nearest emergency room.

3. *Go to your nearest emergency department:* If you are not under the care of a health care provider, or if your regular therapist or physician is unavailable, going to your nearest ER will ensure that you are taken care of immediately.

This chapter covered the symptoms of various postpartum mental health problems. If you are having symptoms yourself, you now understand that these symptoms are part of a well-defined illness. Hopefully you do not feel that you are alone or that you are going crazy because of how you feel. And, in the chapters ahead, you will learn how to help yourself feel better, and how to get the help you need to move out of this dark experience and to stay well.

Chapter 4
Start by Helping Yourself

This chapter will cover techniques that you can use on your own to help you get through PPD and PPA. Whether you are pregnant and at risk of PPD or PPA, or if you are already suffering, there is something here for you. These are powerful tools that you can start using right now. If you keep an open mind and are willing to dedicate some time to using these techniques, you can start to feel better quickly.

The chapter starts by teaching you how to talk to yourself in a healthier way. By becoming aware of negative or anxious thoughts you will learn how to address them. You will also learn how to better care for yourself through eating, exercising, and getting more sleep. Yes, you read that correctly: You can and should get more sleep. Let's get started.

Tuning in to Your Thoughts

If you have recently had a baby and you think you have PPD or PPA, there are bound to be grim, frightening, and self-deprecating thoughts going through your mind right now. It is also likely that you are blaming yourself for how you are functioning, feeling, or caring for your baby. Thoughts like these are increasing your anxiety levels and making you feel even worse.

To start feeling better, you need to address the unhelpful thoughts about yourself, your baby, and the world. Why is this essential? When you are depressed or really anxious, you see the world in a particularly pessimistic way that perpetuates your anxiety or depression. For example, when Jean was depressed, she concluded that her friend didn't like her because her friend cancelled a play date. You can see how if Jean continues thinking this way, it is bound to make her feel sadder and more depressed and to withdraw from her friends. This is the vicious cycle of depression. So, by being aware of the negative way you are thinking about yourself and your situations, you can start to make changes that will help you feel better.

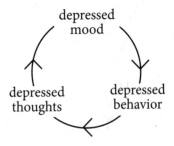

Although it is tempting to ignore the negative thoughts with the hope that they will disappear, this does not usually work. The longer you continue to have such thoughts, the more likely you will be to buy into them, and the more likely they will maintain your depressed or anxious state. Or, you might not even be aware that you have unhealthy, negative thought patterns. After all, these are mostly automatic and occur unconsciously.

But once you become aware of how you see the world and how your outlook may be contributing to your depression or anxiety, you can train yourself to react differently. Studies have shown that when depressed people can be optimistic or shift their thinking along more positive paths, they do really well and move toward recovery. This may take some hard work, but it will help you to be more resilient in the face of depression.

> The ways you are thinking about the world can be part of the cause, as well as a symptom, of your depression or anxiety—and you can change these thoughts.

The idea that your thoughts influence your feelings is based on cognitive behavioral therapy (CBT). The theory behind CBT is that if you have negative thoughts about yourself or a situation, it will translate into negative feelings, such as depression and anxiety, and behaviors that reflect and reinforce depression. Therefore, by changing how you think about something, you can change how you feel and act. Cognitive behavioral therapy is an excellent and well-established treatment for depression in general, and you can make use of some key CBT techniques right here. You can control how you feel by changing how you think.

There are several common negative thinking patterns, formally known as cognitive distortions or negative cognitions that arise in women with PPD or PPA. In his well-known guide, *The Feeling Good Handbook*, Dr. David Burns outlines the 10 most common cognitive distortions that people with depression have. I will explain each of these, with an example that you may relate to, as well as some things to think about if you relate to these patterns. Read through the examples below. Think about which patterns you use and how these patterns are affecting your mood and behavior. Jot down your findings.

All-or-Nothing Thinking

Definition: You think in extreme ways or see the world in black and white with no consideration for the large gray zone, which makes up most of life.

Example: You were feeling exhausted and you asked your best friend, who has been really helpful, to come help take care of the baby so you can have a nap. She said she would come over, but changed her plans at the last minute. You decide that you are never going to speak to her again, and that your friendship is over.

A more balanced approach: Try to understand and live in the gray zone. Relationships may involve upset and disappointment, but that does not mean that they should end. It is totally understandable why you feel let down and upset, and you have every right to tell your friend how you feel, but don't jump to the extreme conclusion in a moment of anger and decide that you need to end a relationship that has mostly been very supportive and helpful.

> If you often use words like "always" or "never" or "completely," you may have all-or-nothing thinking.

Overgeneralization
Definition: You think that if one negative thing happens, then only negative things will continue to happen to you.

Example: Yesterday, your mother told you that you did not dress your baby appropriately for the weather, so you think that everything you are doing with the baby must be wrong and incompetent.

A more balanced approach: Maybe you made one mistake with your child, but this does not mean that everything you do is wrong. Remember, learning to care for a child is an endless process. You will make some mistakes, but that is okay. (And also, don't take others' feedback too personally or literally. Sometimes others' ideas and standards are different from yours. Stick to your guns!) Forgive yourself for the mistakes you make, learn from them, and move on.

Mental Filter
Definition: You ignore the positives of a situation and focus on the negatives.

Example: You took your baby to a music class and everything seemed to be going really well. Then your baby began to cry uncontrollably and you could not soothe her, so you left the class promptly and concluded that this was a "total disaster" and that you won't return to this class.

A more balanced approach: The baby really seemed to enjoy most of the class, then she got upset, or tired, or overstimulated. Babies cannot tell us how they feel, so they cry. And they sometimes cry a lot, especially when we don't want them to! But just because a situation did not turn out the way you had hoped (which can often be the case with a newborn), you can still call it a success. It is important not to let the negatives discolor the whole experience. There will be plenty of good and some not-so-good in most mothering situations and in life!

Disqualifying the Positive

Definition: You undermine your own positive attributes and qualities.

Example: Your partner brings home flowers for you and tells you that you are doing a wonderful job as a mother. You immediately list all of the things you are not doing well and talk about your shortcomings.

A more balanced approach: Think about all the amazing things you are doing as a mother and how much you have learned. Say "thank you" when others give you compliments. Before underscoring your less desirable qualities, dwell on the positives. You will feel so much better.

Jumping to Conclusions

Definition: You assume that others see you in a critical or negative light.

Example: You decide to join a group for new mothers. You look around the room and instantly think that all the other mothers are "total naturals" because they look so happy and are breast-feeding their babies. You are convinced that they think you are a lousy mom when you pull out a bottle to feed your baby.

A more balanced approach: Just because other women choose different feeding methods does not mean that they are being critical of you, or that you have made the wrong decision for yourself. Watch when you make assumptions about how others are thinking or feeling, and particularly about how they perceive you. Chances are that others are not even focusing on you at all.

Magnification and Minimization

Definition: When something negative happens, you overemphasize it while discounting your positive accomplishments.

Example: You were able to clean your house, do three loads of laundry, and bathe and feed your baby, but you did not have time to finish making dinner before your partner got home. You feel like every other woman can do *all* of these things, so you should be able to as well. You worry that your partner will be disappointed with you.

A more balanced approach: It sounds like you have exceedingly high expectations of yourself and that you are discounting the extensive list of things that you are doing while zooming in on the one thing you have not completed. Make a list of what you have done today or this week to appraise realistically your accomplishments and see how effective you *really* are.

Emotional Reasoning

Definition: You base your view of a situation, of yourself, or of others on how you are feeling rather than on reality.

Example: You have been feeling depressed since your baby was born, so you think that you should not have had a baby.

A more balanced approach: You are depressed and you have PPD, but this is *not* evidence of your inability to mother. Instead of saying "I feel, therefore, it is …," you need to look at evidence other than your emotions in order to draw conclusions. Again, make a list of your strengths as a mother. Also practise being gentle with yourself—you are depressed and need to realize that this is coloring how you evaluate yourself and the world around you.

"Should" Statements
Definition: You give yourself a list of things you "should" do and feel badly if you do not do them.

Example: You tell yourself that you "should" register your baby for sign language classes or you "should" be reading more books to your child, or you "should" fit into your pre-pregnancy jeans already. These "should" statements often reflect unrealistic or excessive demands of yourself. You dwell on your perceived shortcomings and feel badly.

A more balanced approach: There are so many things that "experts" as well as friends and family tell you to do as a mother. You want to do some of these, but you cannot do it all. Be realistic about setting your limits for your baby and for yourself. Not doing some of these things doesn't mean you are a bad or neglectful mother. Decide and list your own values and priorities.

Labeling and Mislabeling
Definition: You call yourself negative names.

Example: You leave your daughter with a babysitter while you go to the gym. You tell yourself that you are a "neglectful" mother and are really "selfish" for taking time to care for yourself.

A more balanced approach: Exercise is a healthy and proactive thing to do, and every woman needs to take time for herself. Plus, it is good for your baby to learn to be comfortable with other caregivers. Watch how easily you criticize yourself for being selfish when you do something for yourself.

Personalization

Definition: You criticize and blame yourself if things go badly in situations that are largely beyond your control.

Example: You have had a really rough night when your baby would not sleep for more than 20 minutes at a time and would not settle down, so you tell yourself: "I must be doing something wrong. I will never figure out how to care for this baby. I am not cut out to be a mother."

A more balanced approach: There will be many situations as a mom when hindsight will tell you how you might have done something differently. Life is full of challenging situations. When you encounter a rough time, it does not mean that you are at fault or are a deficient person. Challenges will arise. It helps to deal with the situation and not blame yourself.

Some of these thinking styles are keeping your depression and anxiety alive and well. Although you may not know exactly which ones you use, you can start to monitor your thinking and how it influences your feelings. Pretend that you are carrying around a little tape recorder in your pocket and try to catch yourself when you say things like "always" or "never" or "nothing" or other sweeping, negative generalizations about yourself and your abilities. Or when you feel very badly about yourself or a given situation, examine your thoughts at that moment and try to assess whether or not they reflect distorted thinking. If you find yourself saying some of the things described in the examples above, this is a good indicator of your unhelpful patterns.

When you catch yourself, write down your findings. Notice the situations that upset or anger you. Next, write down the thoughts that occur to you in the tricky situation. Then note your mood. After that, write down a more balanced and less self-critical way to deal with the situation. This way you will be able to observe yourself and your reactions, and then talk yourself into new ways of coping with hard situations instead of jumping into thinking modes that prolong your depression.

It can be tricky to recognize what you are doing and to come up with a balanced way to assess the situation, but try it! If you need to bounce ideas off someone, talk to your partner, family members or friends for feedback. Sometimes those who are close to us can see our patterns more clearly than we can. You may also find it helpful to seek talk therapy to address your thinking patterns, which will be discussed in the coming chapters.

Here is a way to record your thoughts and feelings:

Situation: _____

_____

Negative Thoughts: _____

_____

Mood: _____

_____

Balanced Thoughts: _____

_____

It is important to remember that we all use some of these patterns, to varying degrees, at different times. If we are not depressed, we can usually minimize our negative thoughts and put them in perspective. However, when someone suffers from depression, these thinking styles can take on a life of their own. It becomes hard to shake the negativity. Remember that this is your depression talking, not you.

> While you are struggling with PPD and caught in a vicious cycle of self-defeating thoughts and harsh feelings, here are some positive things to remember:
>
> 1. My thoughts about myself, my baby, and my future are distorted by my postpartum depression.
>
> 2. I am taking charge of my PPD and helping myself feel better.
>
> 3. I feel this way now, but I will not feel this way forever.
>
> 4. I am not a bad mother or a bad person.
>
> 5. This is not my fault.
>
> You can copy down these statements and read them to yourself when you are feeling particularly down and depressed. Use them as a reminder and a helpful way to stop your vicious thought cycle.

How to Combat Anxiety

As discussed in Chapters 2 and 3, women with postpartum anxiety disorders may have some of the same thinking styles as women who are primarily depressed, but they also have a particular way of thinking that perpetuates their anxious symptoms. Now you will learn what you can do to combat your anxious thoughts and feelings.

Just to recap, there are three major components to anxiety that need to be addressed: First, women with anxiety often have "what if" or catastrophic thinking; they worry that something terrible will happen in the future. Second, they fear they will be unable to handle a potential crisis. And third, they get awful

physical symptoms. Let's talk about how to manage each part
of the anxiety cycle. You can use these techniques at any time
in any place. They don't cost a thing. And they can be used
whether your anxiety level is low or high.

Step 1: Managing the Anxious Thoughts

1. Catch yourself when you feel threatened or
   vulnerable. Write down the details of the situation
   or your worries.
2. Consider the evidence to support why the situation
   may be hard or your worries are justified.
3. Consider the evidence to support why the situation
   is not as bad as you think.

**Step 2: Improving Your Confidence So That You Can
Cope with a Difficult Situation**

1. Remind yourself that you can cope with hard
   situations if you need to.
2. List some challenges you have faced.
3. List how you coped with these challenges.
4. Make a list of people you can call if you need help.
   (For example, call your partner, call a friend who
   also has a newborn baby to seek reassurance, call
   your mother, call the pediatrician, call a help line,
   or reread this section.)

Step 3: Managing the Physical Symptoms of Anxiety

 • Relaxation exercise

Progressive muscular relaxation can help you relax when you
feel very nervous. You can do this lying down or sitting up.
The goal is to tense and relax all the muscles from your head to
your toes. Start at the top of your body, tighten your forehead

for five seconds, then relax it for 10 seconds; squeeze your eyes closed for five seconds, then relax them for 10 seconds; tighten your mouth for five seconds, then relax it for 10 seconds, etc. Continue to do this for all the major muscles in your body, down to your toes.

There are many other similar body-relaxation exercises. If you know and like another one, do it when you feel anxious.

- Deep breathing

This is a very simple and straightforward technique to help you to relax when you feel tense. By slowing down your breathing, you will feel much calmer. Breathe in for four seconds, then out for four seconds for at least four minutes. Breathe gently.

- Visualize the anxiety

This approach is particularly helpful if you have panic attacks or episodes of intense anxiety that overwhelm you. The goal of this exercise is not to fight the anxiety but observe it, let it happen to you, then let it pass over you. Here's how:

1. When you start to feel your anxiety increasing or symptoms developing, visualize the anxiety as a wave.
2. Watch the wave come toward you.
3. Feel the wave wash over you.
4. Watch the wave get smaller and recede.

- Distraction

Instead of focusing on your anxious feelings and symptoms, this approach encourages you to forget about them and turn your attention elsewhere. There are many ways to do this: You can look out the window and carefully observe your surroundings; you can change activities; you can try counting things; or you can tell yourself a pleasant story. See what works for you.

The goal of these techniques is not to fight the anxiety or to get upset with yourself for feeling anxious or to start calling yourself names. The goal is to relax your mind and body when you feel highly anxious. For example, let's meet Audrey and look at how she managed her anxiety.

Audrey was a new mother who came to see me when she was three weeks postpartum because she felt that her worries were out of control. Her anxiety began when her baby was one week old and sounded very congested. Even though the pediatrician told Audrey that it was normal "newborn mucus," she was still very worried. Then, when the baby was two weeks old, she developed a rash in her mouth and was spitting up a lot. Audrey took her baby to the hospital and was reassured that the baby had a mild case of thrush and that the spitting up was nothing to be worried about. However, Audrey did not feel reassured. She constantly worried about more germs coming into her house and about her baby getting sick. She worried that the doctors were missing an ominous diagnosis and that the baby was indeed very ill. She also worried that she could not be alone with her baby for fear of something terrible happening that she would not be able to cope with. Here are Audrey's anxiety management exercises.

Step 1: Managing the Anxious Thoughts (Consider the evidence.)

1. Whenever my baby has a slight symptom of an illness, I feel worried. I cannot stop myself from thinking that the worst will happen. I get sweaty and edgy and cannot sleep.
2. My baby has had some minor health issues that have required treatment and care.

3. There has been nothing seriously wrong with my baby. She is generally very healthy and is thriving. Plus, I have a great pediatrician whom I can call if there is a problem.

Step 2: Improving Your Confidence So That You Can Cope with a Difficult Situation (List the challenges that you have managed well.)

Challenge 1

1. My mother had pneumonia a few years ago.
2. I took her to the hospital and was very calm. I learned how to navigate the health care system to help my family.

Challenge 2

1. I lost my job last year.
2. I felt very depressed and anxious after this happened. I opened up to my husband and to my mother about how I felt, and I began to feel much better over time. I also started doing yoga, which really helped me to feel calmer and healthier. With help from my good friend, I developed a plan to find another job. I got a job that I love.
3. If I am concerned about my baby, I can call my mom, my pediatrician, or the local health line.

Step 3: Managing the Physical Symptoms of Anxiety

I can do my relaxation exercises, yoga stretches, and practise deep breathing.

All of the techniques discussed are portable and effective, but they may require some practice. Try them a few times before judging whether they work or not. You may want to experiment to see which approach works best for you. Feel free to use a combination of strategies, or try different ones at different times. Note your anxiety before and after doing these exercises to see how effective they are.

Managing Your Expectations

Motherhood is a lightning rod for fantasies. Many women have elaborate and often unrealistic fantasies about what they will be like as a mother, about the experience of being a mother, and what their baby will be like. At the best of times, if reality does not live up to fantasy, this can be upsetting. When you have PPD, these disappointments can be really devastating. Because, as discussed above, depression and anxiety can skew your perspective and give you a negative slant on the world, the misconceptions or disappointments that you may experience as a mother hit harder and can make you feel worse. They can perpetuate your depressed or anxious state and keep you in a negative cycle: You feel down on yourself for not living up to "mothering standards," you feel depressed, and then you feel worse about yourself.

These are issues that come up time and again for women I see with PPD or PPA. I am including them here to help you help yourself. I am offering you another way to think about things that often upset new moms with depression or anxiety. While there are not always things you can do to change these expectations or change your experience, being aware of what you are feeling and how you're feeling let down can go a long way toward feeling relief. Plus, you will see you are not alone in your struggles.

You Don't Have to Love Your Baby Right Away

Many women with PPD have trouble feeling any positive feelings at all and they do not immediately fall madly in love with their babies. This does not mean that there is anything wrong with them.

Understand that depression is getting in the way of feeling love for and connectedness with your baby. That bond will strengthen as your PPD heals. Also, remember that not all women bond immediately with their babies.

For now, forgive yourself and be patient. Remind yourself that your thoughts and feelings are colored by your illness and that you are getting help. Try to remove the layer of guilt on top of the hard feelings you are already having. As tough as it may be, accept that this is where you are right now, but know that things will get better. You are not having these thoughts because you are a bad person or an unfit mother.

In the meantime, you can also work on developing a connection with your baby. I will discuss some practical tips for doing this in Chapter 10.

You Will Redefine "Normal"

Many new mothers have great expectations about how much they will love being a mother and enjoy a new lifestyle. They look forward to hours of playing and playdates, being off work, taking long walks, sitting in cafés, and traveling with their newborns. Then reality strikes. Many women find it difficult to leave the house with their baby for the first while, they find they have no time to relax, and feel too frazzled to sit in a café and sip a latte.

When the reality of mothering a newborn does not jive with your fantasy, this can be disappointing and frustrating. Diapers, poops, constant feeding, sore breasts, and exhaustion come to define motherhood for you. And your struggles with these might outweigh any joy you are experiencing.

Expect the first few months to be an adjustment period, and realize that it will take time to adjust to the "new normal" that is your life. This does not mean you will *never* be able to take long, leisurely walks or travel with ease. (Again, monitor your extreme thinking habits.) But the ease is not likely to come immediately, and will take time to achieve.

By *taking each day as it comes* and not thinking that the rest of motherhood is going to be onerous and exhausting just because today may be, you will feel much better. Honestly—I know that this sounds like a cliché, but please try it. I say it all the time to my patients and although their eyes gloss over when they first hear it, this reminder has been very helpful.

Allison told me: "When you said, 'Take one day at a time,' I thought you were spewing clichés from a new age book. But then when I went home and felt overwhelmed by my baby throughout a really bad night. Those words popped into my head and got me through the night. I was able to start the next morning with a fresh emotional slate and actually enjoy my day."

> Take one day at a time ... for real!

Embrace Ambivalence

Many new mothers are surprised by the array of extreme emotions they experience. They may sometimes feel very happy, but may also feel frustrated, overwhelmed, and regretful. Some women get scared at the slightest hint of a less-than-joyous feeling about motherhood. Be assured that ambivalent feelings are totally normal.

The problem for moms with PPD or PPA is that the feelings of ambivalence are often harder to tolerate because if you have PPD or PPA, chances are that your guilt is running rampant. To add any less-than-positive feelings to this mix feels terrible and your guilt shoots through the roof.

But whether or not you are suffering from PPD, know that you will have some less charitable feelings. Accept these and realize they are normal. Do not judge yourself for your feelings. Also, when you are feeling badly about motherhood or about your baby, pause and take note of the situation that is triggering these feelings. Take note of your state of mind, your level of exhaustion, and the help and support you are (or are not) getting. These are important things to examine, especially when motherhood feels too hard. Chances are you can make some changes in one of these areas, which may help you ease your burden and feel better.

Whenever Paige started to feel overly frustrated with her baby, she knew it was a signal that she had to get some time for herself. She asked her husband to take over baby care duties for a few hours and went to a coffee shop to read magazines. When Paige came back, she felt revived and much less burdened.

Rather than judging yourself harshly for feeling ambivalent, accept these feelings as part of the journey and make changes where possible. Talking to someone you trust about your feelings may also be helpful.

> Start to accept ambivalent feelings: It's normal, it's motherhood!

Let Yourself Learn: Be a Student of Motherhood

Particularly for the perfectionists among us who have PPD or PPA, not knowing all the ins and outs of baby care from day one is totally unnerving. But every expectant and new mother needs to let herself evolve as a parent. You need to be prepared to *not* know how to do things and you must remember that you will learn how to manage your baby in time. I know, easier said than done. This is usually a tremendous challenge for women with PPD or PPA, but rest assured that you will adapt and evolve as a parent. I once heard a very wise person say: "When a baby is born, so is a mother." This is a good saying to keep in mind. You are learning how to be a mother and, like learning everything else, this process takes time.

To make the process easier, try to accept that you do not know it all. At the same time, you can educate yourself by talking to other women who seem to share your outlook and approach to parenting. Read books, find good Web sites, attend talks, etc. To help you with this, there are many resources listed at the back of this book. But remember, much of your learning will be done "on the job" and you will develop your own confidence and style in time.

Stop Trying to Please

Try to let go of others' expectations of you or your perception of what others expect you to do as a new mother. Chances are that if you are doing this now, you are practised in looking to others for guidance or validation. You are not alone—many women are experts in this field. And with PPD or PPA, you likely feel sapped of your own confidence or you are having trouble making decisions for yourself, so you are even more prone to seeking advice and validation from others. This is all right to a certain extent if others can provide helpful advice and support, but if it causes you to feel even more guilty and incompetent than you already feel with PPD or PPA, then changes must be made.

There are two ways to deal with this. First, try to distance yourself from those who are giving you too much unwanted and unhelpful advice, or politely request that they stop with the advice giving or meddling. Second, talk with them about their expectations.

Natalie was having a very hard time breastfeeding her baby.

She tried everything, but was feeling very anxious and was heading toward a depression. She desperately wanted to stop breastfeeding. However, Natalie was terrified that her husband would be very critical of her and deeply disappointed with her decision not to continue. When Natalie actually asked him what his hopes and expectations were regarding breastfeeding, he could not have been more supportive of her decision to stop. He saw how stressful and anxiety-provoking nursing had become. She felt free to make a choice once she knew he supported her.

This is not always possible to do, but it can be a huge relief if you can clarify your feelings with other people. If you have a long history of relying on others' reactions and opinions of you, this may be something to explore with a professional therapist.

Giving up Control to Gain Peace of Mind

At the risk of sounding like a broken record, now is the time when you need to lessen your expectations of what you can accomplish in a day and about the state of order in your home. Try not panic as your "to do" list lengthens and your house looks disheveled. The newborn period is a time when your focus will necessarily shift from the tidiness of your home to caring for your baby. I know this can be a hard pill to swallow, particularly for a perfectionist, but you simply won't be able to get as much done as you usually do. To ease your guilt and stress, try not to dwell on this or feel badly about yourself for having to change the pace at which you do things.

Again, by reminding yourself that this stage is not forever, you may feel less overwhelmed and more accepting. When you have a newborn baby and are depressed or anxious, it is essential to minimize your expectations of yourself and your accomplishments *for the time being.* You will just feel down on yourself and more overwhelmed if you try to uphold your pre-baby and non-depressed standards and expectations.

If letting things slide increases your anxiety, try asking other people to help you out. If there is ever a time for you to learn to accept help, this is it. I will discuss how to do this and what to ask others to do in the pages ahead.

Comparison Shopping: Every Mom and Every Baby Are Different!

It is hard not to compare your baby to other children or to the babies you read about in books. Everyone does this, but it can be a particular issue for women with PPD or PPA. When you are depressed and telling yourself that "Everyone else is doing things so well and so easily while I can't do anything right," you get caught up looking over your shoulder and being self-critical and envious.

Not only do new moms compare babies, they also compare themselves to other mothers: "Can you believe that Michelle was already wearing her old jeans when her baby was only three weeks old?" "I should be more like Paula and make all of my own baby food and use only organic produce." "How can Melissa already be back at the gym?" "Sandra already has enrolled her baby in preschool." The list goes on and on.

How to Minimize Your Comparisons

When you get caught up in comparisons, stop yourself in your tracks. First, see what you are doing and how it is making you feel about yourself. Second, think about and make a list of the things you love about your baby and like about yourself as a mother and what you think you are doing really well. This exercise is not meant for you to continue to compare yourself with others, but for you to stop and take stock of your strengths. You might feel that these are limited right now, but dig deep or ask someone close to you to help you with this list.

Just as your baby is a unique individual who will do things within a unique time frame, so are you. This is not to say that you can't learn from other mothers' experiences or styles, or admire qualities in other babies. In fact, other moms can be your best friends and invaluable resources about child rearing, but admiring and learning from others is very different from feeling deficient and envious. When your own strengths are at the forefront of your mind, it is much harder to condemn yourself.

Easier Said Than Done

Yes, I know. I often hear, "Dr. Dalfen, I know that what you're telling me makes sense, but I just don't know how to make these changes." First, I am not asking you to make all of these changes at once and immediately. You will recall that the first steps to take involve observing yourself, getting to know yourself better, and understanding what triggers you. If you can do only that, you are already doing so much. Psychological changes often take time and occur slowly, and it is also likely that you are trying to unlearn old patterns and habits that you have had for many years. But stay hopeful and know that they will happen.

Remember, just because we are talking about your emotions and thoughts does not mean that you are at fault or to blame for having PPD or PPA; these examples are simply some of the personal things you *can* take control of.

Although some people find that these things are best discovered with a professional therapist—and I will discuss the importance of psychotherapy in the next chapter—I encourage you to start this journey now, on your own.

And you can always use a variety of techniques and treatments to get better and stay well. If you try the strategies outlined in this chapter, you will be on your way to feeling better and to addressing the thoughts and feelings that underlie your depression or anxiety.

I know all of this can sound and feel overwhelming, but these strategies can expedite the healing process and help you take control of your recovery.

Caring for Yourself

In this section, I will discuss how you can take control of your sleep and your eating habits, as well as making some other simple changes that will help yourself feel better.

Sleep and PPD

You are likely up to feed your newborn babe every one to three hours throughout the night. Even if your baby is sleeping with you or right next to you, these constant awakenings are disruptive. Night after night of disturbed sleep can get to you (and I see you nodding in agreement). Some women are able to fall back to sleep quickly after waking up to feed their baby, but most women with PPD or PPA find that they have trouble falling asleep and staying asleep, as their minds tend to start racing and their bodies are unable to relax. Some women with postpartum problems begin to fear nighttime and are consumed with the prospect that they will soon be awakened, so not only do they have poor-quality sleep, but sleep becomes a tremendous source of anxiety and dread, which worsens sleep. Another vicious cycle.

As you are well aware, lack of sleep can make everything feel worse and can magnify symptoms of depression or anxiety. You will be thrilled to hear that sleep patterns, or lack thereof, are one of the first things to be addressed when treating PPD or PPA.

> Making changes to your sleep habits often goes a long way toward improving your mood and reducing your anxiety.

Here are several sleep strategies that you can try:

1. Increase the length of your stay in the hospital after the baby is born.
Some hospitals offer extended postpartum stays to women who are at high risk of developing PPD. At the hospital, there are trained nurses who can care for your baby while you take a few extra hours to sleep in this crucial recovery time. And there are even sleeping pills for those women who just cannot find the calm necessary for sleep. A lengthier hospital stay can be a tremendous help in getting you on the right track. There is some research data to show that increasing the amount of time a woman can spend in the hospital postpartum, up to about five days, often goes a long way toward preventing a postpartum mental health episode.

Ask your obstetrician or midwife if your local hospital has this option. If you are at high risk, and if this is available to you, go for it.

2. How to get the rest you need at home.
Getting a decent amount of good-quality nighttime sleep is essential for women with postpartum depression and anxiety disorders. I cannot emphasize this enough. Improving night-time sleep can often avert a serious episode of illness and dramatically improve existing symptoms, but you cannot do

this alone. You need to enlist the help of your partner, family, and friends.

Of course you will want to be close to your baby in these first amazing days, and you will. But a good night's sleep is incredibly important for you and your continued ability to feel good and strong throughout the postpartum period, so don't hold back when it comes to asking for help. At least six hours of nighttime sleep seems to be the key for women with PPD. Having a partner, parent, or friend close by whom you can trust to care for your baby while you rest will give you both the time and the peace of mind needed to sleep soundly.

Some women have a hard time falling asleep if they can hear their baby fussing or making any noises at all, which is perfectly natural, but don't be afraid to really make this brief period about your rest. If you are needed, your "night nurse" will come and wake you, so give yourself permission to kiss your baby goodnight and pop in some earplugs or move to a quiet room—it is for the best for both of you.

Let your partner get a piece of the action: If you are in a relationship, the first step is to have a frank conversation with your partner and ask him or her to help you with the night feedings and baby care. There are various ways to make this happen. Listed below are several creative scheduling options. You can review these with your partner and settle on the one that is most suitable for your family life, considering your work schedules and natural sleep habits.

Divide the Night in Half

If your partner works outside of the home and has a nine-to-five workday, it is still possible for him or her to help with nighttime feeding. Remember, you are in this together and there is no reason why you have to be the only one who is sleep deprived. Although it is difficult to continue to work outside of the home when you have a newborn, it is vital for your partner to help out so that you do not shoulder the entire burden alone. You can both acknowledge that it is hard to work a full day while feeling tired from the night before, but also take comfort in knowing that this is not forever. You might both be tired in the short term, but helping you get sufficient sleep will go a long way toward averting depression, which will ultimately make you a better and more capable mother and partner.

A great way to do this is to divide the night into two shifts. Often it works well if you go to sleep very early after dinner and after feeding the baby, around 7-8 p.m. At that time, your partner can take over baby duty for the next six or seven hours while you sleep soundly. At 1-2 a.m., you can relieve your partner. (Of course, you can adjust the start and stop times of each person's shift to suit your needs and schedules.)

This strategy works well if your partner needs to get up to go to work each morning. With this plan, you can at least get one decent chunk of high-quality nighttime sleep in a 24-hour period and, hopefully, even more.

Some women say that they just can't fall asleep that early, or they need some wind-down time, or want to spend that evening time with their partner or with their other kids. Remember, you don't have to take an all-or-nothing approach to this. You don't have to do it every night of the week if it feels like you are giving up too much. Try it on some nights and not on others, and note how you feel. But again, it is very important during this brief newborn period that you get rest and sleep well, particularly if you have PPD or PPA.

Alternate Nights

Some couples find that their schedules permit them to take on alternating nights of child-care responsibilities. This means that you know you will be up and caring for the baby on Monday night, but that you will be able to sleep well on Tuesday night when the other parent takes over the responsibilities. If your partner works until late at night or does shift work, you may find that this strategy is best.

Divide the Day in Half

Dividing the 24-hour day into two shifts is a particularly good option when both you and your partner are at home. This means that you may divide the day into two segments, where one adult is responsible for one entire shift, while the other adult can sleep. One couple divided the day into two 7 a.m.-7 p.m. shifts. Since the mom, Gabriella, had a history of PPD and needed to sleep well at night, and her husband, Marcus, was off work for a while and was a night owl, this schedule worked well. Gabriella went to sleep at 7 p.m. and was able to sleep all night. Marcus was in charge of baby care while Gabriella slept. Then, between 7 a.m. and 7 p.m., Marcus slept while Gabriella looked after the their baby.

Get Outside Help

If your partner is unable to help with the nighttime baby care, ask a reliable family member or friend to help you out. Even if someone cannot help you every night, getting help on some nights is better than nothing.

Erika had a very generous mother who offered to have Erika, her husband, and their newborn daughter stay at her house once or twice each week. The mother took care of the baby through the night so that both Erica and her husband could sleep well. This plan really helped to relieve Erica's depressive symptoms, even after just a few nights of improved sleep.

How Can I Sleep and Feed My Baby?

There are a few options:

1. If you are bottle-feeding, then it will be a seamless transition to have your partner, parent, or another support look after the baby while you sleep.

2. If you are breastfeeding, you can pump breast milk and put it in a bottle so that your child can still receive your milk while being fed by someone else.

3. If you choose to only breastfeed, then you can certainly start out breastfeeding through the night by having your support or night nurse bring the baby to you for feeds and then taking your babe to change the diaper and help him or her settle back to sleep. But if you choose to breastfeed exclusively, it is important to be flexible. If, after a few days, depressive or anxious symptoms seem to be worsening or not improving at all, maybe it is time to relax the need to exclusively feed at the breast.

I know how important and personal a choice it is to decide to breastfeed or bottle-feed, but if you are dealing with depression or anxiety, you will have to be as flexible as possible in these choices, in order to accommodate your own very important needs right now. Perhaps you are totally set on breastfeeding exclusively, and it is hard for you to imagine anyone else feeding your child from a bottle. Remember that you can pump milk so your baby will still get the breast milk you'd like him or her to have. Though it isn't your perfect scenario, or the way you dreamed it would be, it is a compromise that allows you to get the uninterrupted sleep you need in order to be a good parent in other essential ways and to care for your health. Often women with PPD or PPA feel very anxious about not doing things well, so they find it especially difficult to change paths with regard to feeding, but your role as a parent is multifaceted—your baby needs many different things from you, including love, patience, laughter, and a watchful eye. In order to do your best in all of these roles, some of your ideas and practices regarding breast-feeding may need to be loosened and made flexible.

Hire a Night Nurse

Hiring a night nurse to care for your newborn has become a very popular trend, with good reason. Unfortunately, this can be a very expensive option, but if you can afford it, it is worthwhile, especially for those at risk of postpartum depression and anxiety. A night nurse will come to your home every night, usually around 8 or 9 p.m. He or she will take care of your baby throughout the night to allow you to maximize your sleep time. If you choose to continue to breastfeed around the clock, your baby will be brought to your bed for you to nurse, and then you can go back to sleep right away. You can hire a night nurse to come for as many or as few days as you want, depending on your financial resources and need.

Some women find that no matter what they try, they simply can't get to sleep. In some instances, sleep medication may be needed for the short term. Medications, their side effects, safety, and duration will be discussed in detail in Chapter 7.

3. Work to Improve Your Baby's Sleep

Of course, the million-dollar question is "How can I get my baby to sleep better?" A full discussion of baby sleep methods is beyond the realm of this book, but please see the Resources section at the back of this book for useful Web sites and books. I strongly suggest that you read some of the books recommended or talk to your pediatrician about improving your baby's sleep habits. When your baby sleeps better, this could bring a significant improvement to your mood and well-being. There are sleep-training strategies that often work very well and quickly. You can find a sleep routine that feels comfortable for you and your family. Having a routine in place will also make it easier on your partner or night nurse, as well as your new baby.

4. Take a Nap

Although nighttime has been shown to be the most important time for healthy sleeping, napping during the day can certainly help reenergize you. My patients often balk at this suggestion. They tell me that they just cannot wind down enough during the day to nap when the baby is sleeping. Or, they say that it takes them too long to fall asleep and when they finally do catch some *zzz*'s, the baby wakes up and they wake up feeling disoriented and not refreshed after 20 minutes. Some new moms say that they cannot sleep because they have too much to do and this is the only precious time they have with their other kids, or for themselves, to try to get anything done.

Yes, when you have a newborn, there is a time crunch, to say the least, but napping can help you feel more energetic, less irritable, and more relaxed, so it is worth a little effort if it doesn't come naturally. You don't have to nap every day to realize the benefits, but try it sometimes. Try napping on those days when you feel most exhausted, and experiment with different lengths of time. Some women swear by the 10-minute nap, while others find they feel much better after half an hour. Even if you don't actually fall asleep, resting quietly can be wonderfully restorative and a perfect break from the go-go-go of parenting.

5. Limit Visitors

Once you have your sleep strategy, ensure that nothing comes between you and your pillow. This means that you don't want the doorbell or the phone to ring. Family and friends may be rushing over or calling to share your excitement and to meet the baby, but make sure that your visitors come at a time that is convenient for you. If you are feeling depressed or anxious, you will probably want to limit who you see and who is in your personal space. You have every right to say no to visitors. You can decide *if* people will come over, *who* will come over, and how long they may stay. You can also turn off your phone or keep phone calls really brief. These principles apply both day and night.

If Breastfeeding Is an Issue

If nursing is going well for you, that is fabulous. Keep it up! But for many new moms, breastfeeding is complicated and painful, and is intimately related to the development of PPD and PPA.

As already discussed, it is unclear if having PPD or PPA makes breastfeeding more difficult, or if nursing troubles cause PPD or PPA. Regardless of your initial feeding plan, being flexible with this significant issue is very important.

Here are a few things to consider if you are worrying about nursing and are depressed and anxious about it:

1. Depression or anxiety disorders may be causing you to negatively evaluate your breastfeeding experience or to see nursing problems as insurmountable. You can try to hold on to see if your experience with breastfeeding improves as your mood and anxiety get better.
2. Consult with a lactation consultant for suggestions about how to make breastfeeding work for you. They can often help you learn to feed with ease. Ask your obstetrician, midwife, or pediatrician to refer you to a good lactation consultant.
3. Of course, you are very invested in your chosen feeding method, and may want to breastfeed exclusively, but it is important to avoid all-or-nothing thinking about this. If your baby is losing weight or your depression

and anxiety are worsening, consider the options .
described in the sleep section of this chapter. Consult
your pediatrician if you are concerned about your
baby. But for you, knowing that you do not have to
nurse exclusively or be the only one responsible for
feeding your child can go a long way toward relieving
some stress and anxiety. A happy mom means a happy,
healthy baby.

Eating Well

Trying to eat a well-balanced diet while caring for a newborn
is no mean feat. Grabbing whatever is handy is the norm for a
busy new mom, which often leads to making poor food choices.
Plus, new mothers with PPD or PPA often find that they have
no appetite. However, it is essential to eat healthy foods to
maintain your physical stamina. At first, you may not mind
that your appetite is down and that you are losing your baby
weight, but it is very important to keep eating well. If you are
already suffering from depression or anxiety, and you neglect
to eat or eat too much junk food, your energy, motivation, and
enthusiasm will be even further depleted.

Here are some tips for nutritious eating:

1. Don't forget to eat. You may not have regular mealtimes,
   but eat when you can.
2. Eat a balanced diet and make healthy food choices
   whenever possible. A balanced diet consists of protein
   (meat and fish), carbohydrates (breads, pastas, muffins),
   healthy fats (olive oil, avocado, fish oils), plenty of fruit
   and vegetables, and lots of water.
3. Allow yourself treats in moderation.
4. If you find that no foods seem appealing, stick to foods

that that will give you a good caloric and nutritional bang for your buck. For example, make a yogurt-and-fruit smoothie.

5. Fill your fridge with healthy finger foods or other things that you can eat with one hand while holding or feeding your baby, such as prepared sandwiches or pieces of fruit. Better yet, have someone else fill your fridge!

6. Ask friends and family to bring over meals or snacks. This is a great practical way to ask for help.

7. Take advantage of food-delivery services: Groceries can be ordered online and delivered to your home, and restaurant delivery services are even easier.

8. Drink lots of water. Especially for women who are breastfeeding, it is essential to stay well hydrated and to drink a lot of decaffeinated and nonalcoholic drinks. Water is a great choice and is also vital for energy levels during this period, so drink it as often as possible.

9. Take a multivitamin. This will give you what you may be missing from your diet and will ensure you stay healthy if you are nursing.

10. Consider adding omega-3 fatty acids to your diet. There is emerging data that omega-3 fatty acids may help treat postpartum depression. This is not yet definitive evidence, and it is no substitute for proper treatment. But for now you can eat omega-3-rich foods, such as salmon, flaxseeds, and walnuts.

11. Limit caffeine and alcohol. I suggest you drink very little or no caffeine and alcohol while nursing. Remember that these beverages are dehydrating, so make sure that you drink even more water throughout the day if you consume coffee or alcohol.

Alcohol and Caffeine
Alcohol

There is a complicated relationship between alcohol and depression. Many people who feel down or anxious drink alcohol because it helps them to relax and to feel better for a short while, but alcohol acts as a depressant and can actually make depression worse.

Also, the alcohol that a mother drinks passes into her breast milk and is processed by a newborn baby at very slow rates. High levels of alcohol in breastfed babies have been shown to affect their sleep habits and physical coordination. Alcohol may also change the taste of breast milk and may be a turnoff for your baby. If you choose to drink alcohol while breastfeeding, please be aware that it takes nearly two and a half hours for a 130-pound woman to process one drink! One or two drinks a week while you are nursing may be fine but make sure enough time has passed before nursing so you will not pass alcohol along to your baby. The safest thing is not to expose your baby to any alcohol at all.

Caffeine

Caffeine often triggers anxiety and should be limited or cut out, particularly if you suffer from severe anxiety. Caffeine can also interrupt your sleep patterns and worsen insomnia. Some new moms find that it is easier for them to nap during the day and sleep at night when they avoid caffeine or limit it.

In terms of the safety of caffeine while breastfeeding, caffeine levels in breast milk are very low and unlikely to have an impact on your baby when small or moderate amounts of coffee are consumed. Caffeine reaches a peak level in breast milk after one hour, so if you choose to drink coffee, it is best to do so immediately after the morning feeding, at least one and a half hours before your baby is likely to be hungry again.

In order to be well enough to take care of a little baby, you need to first take care of yourself. Eating enough healthy food and making wise drink choices are important steps in good self-care.

Just Do It: Get Active

We all see the paparazzis' snapshots of celebrities who fit into their tiny jeans two weeks after having a baby, or the unflattering photos with nasty captions of starlets who are called "fat" one month after delivery. These images wreak havoc with the body image of new moms. We get down on ourselves if we do not look like those glamorous skinny new moms. In fact, different women lose weight at different rates and it may take up to one year to lose your baby weight. The best way to stay healthy and to slowly lose the weight that you gained during pregnancy is through a healthy diet and moderate exercise.

Besides, exercise is an important component of treating PPD and PPA. Exercise has been shown to be a useful addition to traditional treatments for depression and anxiety in general. On a physical level, exercise increases endorphins that stimulate the "feel good" center in the brain. You may find that your mind relaxes while you exercise and you feel calm afterwards. Psychologically, being active makes you feel that you are taking charge of your life and your body at a time when they may feel out of your control.

You do not need to run marathons or work out at a gym for two hours to get exercise. You can take a leisurely stroll or go for a bike ride. Do yoga or gentle stretches if that feels best.

Some exercise is better than none. Do what you can, when you can.

You can be active on your own if you have some child-care support, or you can incorporate your baby in an activity. Studies have shown that depressed women who joined "strollercize" classes (walking and running with their baby in the stroller) felt less depressed immediately after they exercised. Most cities have exercise classes and programs for new mothers and their babies. Check around your neighborhood or ask other moms to see what is available. You can also go online or read local papers for more information.

It is important to speak with your doctor or midwife before you start a postpartum exercise regimen. Most women are advised to wait for at least six weeks before they start to exercise, especially following a C-section, but if you had an uncomplicated vaginal birth and are in good shape, you may be able to start sooner. Even if you were not a regular exerciser before, it is a great idea to start now. Start slowly and build up steadily. You can start by going for a 10-minute walk and add more time daily. (If you have severe anxiety or panic attacks, you may need to start exercising really slowly so that you do not feel anxious when you exert yourself.)

If going to the gym or to an exercise class is not your thing, here is a list of activities that also count as exercise:

1. Go for a walk in the park.
2. Go for a bike ride.
3. Go in-line skating.
4. Go for a swim in your local pool.
5. Turn on your TV and dance to a music station for 20 minutes.
6. Jog to do your errands.

Be creative—just start moving!

Getting Out of the House

When people are depressed, they often feel the need to withdraw from the rest of the world. They either feel too tired to go out, worry that others dislike them, or they feel intensely negative and irritated by other people. When you have a newborn baby, it sometimes feels impossible to get out of the house, but getting outside can have a remarkable effect on your state of mind. You will find that going outside, even for a short time each day, will help you feel better. You will feel more connected to the rest of the world, distracted from your own problems, and you may even enjoy some sunshine and socializing.

Get out at least once a day. At first, your outing can be as simple as going to pick up milk or taking your baby for a stroll around the block. As you feel better, you can make plans to meet other people and stay out longer. Don't overdo it, but do try to go out regularly.

> Plan to go out once a day.

Taking Time for Yourself

It seems every self-help book for women talks about this point. Yet, it is so hard for new moms to put this into practice, and it is doubly challenging for those with depression and anxiety. When you do have a few free moments, you are likely to feel guilty about taking time alone.

Please put your guilty feelings or judgments about being "selfish" aside. The more you respect your personal needs and your need for "me time," the better you will feel. Plus, you will be a more energized and happy mom to your baby and a more relaxed partner and friend.

Take time away from everyone else to do what you enjoy, whether it is going for a jog, window-shopping, painting a picture, or writing in your journal while sitting in a coffee shop.

You need to replenish yourself. Doing so will revitalize you, make you feel great, and reconnect you to yourself and your interests. The more regularly you do something for yourself, the better you will feel and the easier it will be to do.

Plan to take some time for yourself, even if it is only one hour, at least once a week. Please, *really* do this.

You know you *really* need to take time for yourself when:

1. You are feeling more frustrated and are yelling at your partner or your other children.

2. Everything annoys you.

3. You feel very impatient.

4. You feel exhausted.

5. You feel more tense and on edge.

6. You have thoughts such as "I'm at the end of my rope."

7. You notice more aches and pains and your body feels stressed.

Stabilize and Simplify Your Life

Although sometimes life takes us to unexpected places at inopportune times, the postpartum period is not the time to make major life decisions, if you can help it. Nor is it a good idea to make these changes when you have depression or anxiety. Your hormones are in flux, and your judgment and views are colored by depression and anxiety. Plus, your body and your life have just been through major changes.

If you can, try to delay moving homes or cities or changing jobs or ending relationships. The more you can stabilize the things that you can control, the better you will feel. Surrounding yourself with some predictability and familiarity can go a long way toward helping you adjust to being a mom.

Now you have a host of powerful tools that you can start using right away: Learning how to be aware of your thoughts and retrain your thinking is an amazingly effective way to manage PPD and PPA. When combined with a few good nights' sleep and some lifestyle adjustments, you will be on the road to health. The next chapter will look at getting professional help and taking part in talk therapy. This is another totally safe and effective treatment that can help you not only to feel better, but also to gain important insight into yourself and your relationship with your new baby: It can have far-reaching positive effects, and may not be at all what you imagine.

Chapter 5
Getting Professional Help

In the previous chapter you learned some techniques to help yourself recover from PPD and PPA. You may be wondering if you need to do anything else to feel better and, if so, which steps to take now. The answer to this question really depends on the severity of your symptoms, how long you have been suffering, and the degree to which your symptoms of depression or anxiety are preventing you from living your life and caring for your baby.

Usually the best and most effective treatment program involves a combination of self-care, professional help, and building your own network of support. Almost all women with PPD or PPA will benefit from seeking professional support. You really can and will get better, and professional help usually speeds up the process. Remember, try not to let the myths about PPD prevent you from getting help and feeling your best. Do not continue to suffer in silence, on your own, when there are many wonderful professionals who can guide you through this time with numerous helpful techniques, strategies, and approaches.

You Need Professional Help If...

- You continue to feel badly despite making some lifestyle changes.
- Your depression and anxiety are getting worse.
- You feel it is really hard to take care of yourself.
- You are having trouble taking care of your baby.
- You are not enjoying motherhood at all.
- You cannot sleep or eat.
- You have thoughts about harming yourself or someone else.

In this chapter, I will discuss who can help you. I will explain which professionals you can turn to and explain each professional's training, and how to find a mental health care provider. In the following chapters, I will discuss the services and care that professionals can offer as part of your treatment plan: talk therapy and medications. This will help you determine which kind of professional and what treatment is best for you.

Who to Turn to for Help

There are various medical and mental health professionals who can help you. It can be confusing to know where to start and who to turn to first. Different types of mental health professionals can help you in different ways. Within each of the mental health disciplines described below, there are people who specialize in treating women with pregnancy and postpartum–related mental health problems. If you can find someone with this expertise in your area, this is a good place to start. You may need to see more than one health care professional to treat your PPD. For example, you may see one person for psychotherapy and another for medication if that is what you want and need, so there may be several people who make up your treatment team.

Here are some professionals who can treat your postpartum issues or who can steer you in the right direction if they cannot help you directly.

Your Family Doctor, Obstetrician, or Midwife

You are likely to come into the most frequent contact with your family doctor, obstetrician, or midwife throughout your pregnancy and in the postpartum period, so this is where you should start looking for help. If you are comfortable speaking with your doctor or midwife about PPD or other postpartum mental health symptoms, these professionals will be very helpful to you. Some family doctors and obstetricians have knowledge about postpartum mental illness and can help you to feel better. Usually, your family doctor, midwife, or obstetrician will refer you to a mental health care professional who specializes in treating women with postpartum problems. I will describe these mental health professionals in the pages ahead. You can also speak with your baby's pediatrician if you are more comfortable with this person.

Psychiatrist

A psychiatrist is a doctor with an MD who has gone to medical school. After completing medical school, psychiatrists complete four more years of special residency training to learn how to care for patients with mental illnesses. Psychiatrists can prescribe medication and practise psychotherapy. Some psychiatrists prefer only to prescribe medication and will refer you to another mental health professional for psychotherapy, while others will provide both types of care.

In some places, you can call a psychiatrist's office directly and make an appointment for yourself. Elsewhere, your family doctor or obstetrician may have to refer you to a psychiatrist. If you have heard about a psychiatrist you would like to see, do not hesitate to call him or her or ask your family physician, obstetrician or midwife to write a referral letter for you.

How to Help Your Doctor Help You:

1. Don't be afraid to tell your doctor that you are feeling depressed or anxious.

2. Don't be shy to take a few more minutes of your doctor's time.

3. Go armed with accurate information about PPD or PPA, and tell your doctor what you think you have.

4. Ask your doctor to refer you to an expert. Although your doctor may be wonderful, you might still need more specialized care for your situation. In many places, there are psychiatrists or mental health professionals who specialize in treating women with pregnancy or postpartum mental health issues. Ask your doctor to refer you to a specialized caregiver in your area. See the Resources section for suggestions.

Psychologist

Psychologists are mental health professionals who have advanced graduate training in the study of the human mind, emotions, and behavior. They usually have an MA or a PhD. While some psychologists focus on research, others are expert psychotherapists and provide talk therapy and counseling. Psychologists cannot prescribe medications in Canada or in most parts of the United States.

Often you can arrange directly to see a psychologist, especially one who is in private practice. Your workplace employee-assistance plan or your insurance company may have several psychologists on their rosters whom you can contact for treatment. Otherwise, you may have to pay directly to see a psychologist.

If the main treatment for your PPD is talk therapy, you will be in very capable hands with a good psychologist.

Social Worker

A social worker is a health professional who has an undergraduate or advanced graduate degree in social work. Social workers are trained to help people and their families with emotional and physical needs and to help find resources in their community, such as housing and financial supports. Many social workers are also well trained and expert therapists. They may be able to provide individual, group, family, or couples therapy.

Some social workers work in hospital settings as part of a health care team, while others have private practices where they offer psychotherapy. Again, if your professional treatment plan consists of talk therapy, a social worker can be an excellent choice for you.

Therapist or Counselor

This is where it gets a bit confusing. Anyone who practises psychotherapy (talk therapy) can call himself or herself a therapist or a counselor. Whenever one of the professionals described above practises psychotherapy, he or she is a therapist or a counselor. Often members of other professions develop expertise in a certain type of psychotherapy or in treating a certain illness. Some nurses, occupational therapists, or physiotherapists pursue training and education to become "psychotherapists." But in some places, anyone can call himself or herself a therapist or a counselor, even if that person has no training whatsoever. Before committing to treatment with a therapist or counselor, you should find out about his or her credentials.

When you are seeking a mental health care professional, here are a few things to ask him or her:

1. What are your credentials and professional training?
2. What is your experience in treating postpartum mental health problems?
3. What type of treatment can you provide?
4. How much does this treatment cost?

How Do I Know If This Is the Right Person for Me?

Once you find someone who can provide you with good care for PPD or PPA, you need to determine if this is a person you will be comfortable working with and talking to, which is very important. Whether someone is practising psychotherapy or prescribing medication, you need to feel at ease and trust the person who is helping you. You need to feel listened to, respected, and understood. There is no way to know how you will react before meeting someone, so make your decision after a couple of meetings with this person. Trust your instincts on this. If you feel awkward or uncomfortable, seek help elsewhere. Also, don't be put off by mental health care if the first professional you see is not right for you. (Again, watch the extreme thinking patterns.)

You have the right to get excellent care that meets your needs. Here is a list to remind you of your rights:

1. You can (and should) ask questions about the treatment and goals.
2. You can ask the health care provider about his or her professional training and experience.
3. You can state your hesitation or fears.
4. You can decline to discuss certain issues or answer certain questions.
5. You can disagree with whoever is treating you.
6. You can end treatment and seek help elsewhere.

But please, if you decide to end treatment with one person, don't delay; find another professional soon so you can keep the ball of progress rolling.

What Will Happen When I Consult a Mental Health Care Provider?

Rachel was really nervous about starting psychotherapy. She worried that she would have to lie on a couch and talk about her childhood.

Callie was afraid that as soon as her first meeting with a psychiatrist was over, she would be locked up in the hospital. A lot of moms with PPD or PPA are scared about what will happen when they see a mental health professional. Let's demystify this process.

1. The Assessment

Any professional you see will want to do a thorough assessment. That means that he or she will ask you questions about your current situation and how you are coping, your symptoms, and your risk factors. He or she will want to know about your past and your family as well as your current relationships. You can review Chapters 2 and 3 and the notes you made about your own risk factors and symptoms and bring these to the first meeting.

The more information you can provide, and the more details you can recall, the better. Although it may be stressful and embarrassing to open up to someone you don't know, this is the necessary first step in getting good care that can really meet your needs and help you feel better.

2. The Diagnosis and the Plan

Once a professional gets to know you and has enough information, he or she will make a diagnosis and suggest a treatment plan for you. Feel free to mention what you think your diagnosis might be since you have read Chapter 3. And if you have ideas about what you need to feel better, share these thoughts.

There is no exact formula to decide what type of treatment you need once you consult a professional. When you feel a bit down but are still able to live your life as you want to and enjoy your baby most of the time, some of the self-care strategies outlined in the last chapter, as well as psychotherapy, may be all that you need. Generally, if you feel that you are very different from your normal self and that your sadness and worry are taking over, you may need medication as well as therapy. Of course, the idea of taking medication can stir up a lot of fears, so I have devoted an entire chapter to addressing your worries and questions about medications.

Depending on the expertise and profession of the mental health professional you see first, either this person will treat you or will refer you to someone else for the best care for you.

3. Rule out Medical Conditions

As mentioned in Chapter 2, there are some medical conditions that are very similar to PPD and PPA or that have PPD-like symptoms. For this reason, once you have postpartum mental health issues, your family doctor or psychiatrist should do a few blood tests to make sure that you do not have one of these medical conditions. Blood tests should be done for the following: your thyroid levels, hemoglobin, iron, and blood sugar. If you have had other significant medical problems in the past that are flaring up now, you should also see your doctors to monitor your physical health and well-being.

> Before you begin treatment for PPD, get blood work to check your thyroid levels, hemoglobin, iron, and blood sugar.

Where Else Can I Find Help?

1. Experienced Friends and Family Members

Friends and family members who have had PPD or PPA can be phenomenal resources for you. They can help you navigate the medical system and steer you in the right direction whether they are near or far away. If they live close to you, they can give you information about local professionals. If you don't know anyone who had PPD, ask your friends and family if they can suggest a psychiatrist or therapist. A good and experienced professional will be very helpful and the right place to start, even if he or she is not experienced with your particular issues.

2. Hospital Programs for Women with PPD

In several larger cities, there are hospitals with special programs or clinics for women with mental health concerns related to pregnancy and the postpartum period. Contact your local hospitals to see if this type of service is offered and see the Resources section at the back of this book.

Through these programs you will likely meet a psychiatrist or another mental health professional who can help you build a solid treatment plan, and the people who work in that program will become valuable resources for you. They will know the community programs in your area, as well as the various options available within the hospital.

If your local hospital does not have a specialized program, the department of psychiatry at the hospital should be able to inform you about local professionals who can help.

3. Use Other Resources in Your Area

Call any local support groups for women with PPD or mental health issues. They often have a list of good professionals.

Contact professional health care or mental health organizations such as the National Alliance on Mental Illness, the American Psychiatric Association, the Canadian Psychiatric Association, or the Canadian Mental Health Association. These organizations are likely to have information about effective mental health professionals who specialize in treating PPD and PPA.

Please see the Resources section at the end of the book for a complete list of organizations and Web sites that can help you find a good professional.

Here's what to do to get help:

- Talk to your family doctor.
- Talk to your obstetrician or midwife.
- Ask for a referral to a mental health professional.
- Talk to friends or family.
- Call your local hospital.
- Call local mental health organizations.
- Call local health organizations.
- Call local PPD groups.
- Go online: www.postpartum.net and www.postpartum.org have suggestions about how you can find professionals in your area.

No matter where you live, you can get help for PPD or PPA. The next steps are to learn what the professionals can offer you and how different treatments can and will help you get well soon. The next chapter will cover talk therapy and how it can help you through postpartum problems, and Chapter 7 will discuss when medication is appropriate.

Chapter 6
Psychotherapy

Words are, of course, the most powerful drug used by mankind.
—Rudyard Kipling

Psychotherapy, like PPD, has its own myths that often stop women from considering it as an option. While there are studies and scientific research showing that all the forms of therapy discussed in this chapter can be beneficial for treating depression, there are still many fears about seeking this kind of support: "Will it make me look weak? Will it confirm I am crazy? Will it make me dependent on someone else? Will it uncover something I simply don't want to think about or know more about? Will I be comfortable confiding everything to a total stranger? Will it work quickly enough? What will other people say? Does it even work?"

These are common and real concerns that you may have about seeing a therapist, but please don't let these fears stand in your way and don't let the myths about therapy overwhelm or paralyze you. The reality is that you are feeling badly now and that therapy can be a very effective and positive treatment to help you get better. Many other women have participated in psychotherapy to treat their PPD and PPA and found that they felt much better, much stronger, and more confident. Therapy may be the only treatment that you pursue or, as is often the case with PPD or PPA, it may be part of a larger treatment plan that includes personal changes and medication. Not only can psychotherapy help your symptoms now, it can also help you solve some of the issues that have triggered your depression or anxiety. You do not need to continue therapy forever to stay well. It can help you learn a lot about yourself and deal with your PPD or PPA in the short term, and there will most definitely be long-term gain from the process too. I encourage you to give it a try.

> In therapy, you can make short-term and long-term gains.

The essence of talk therapy can be hard for someone who has never done it to understand. The best way to see if psychotherapy is right for you is to find a good therapist and try it out. This chapter will answer some of the most common questions that women with PPD or PPA have about therapy and look at the different kinds of therapy so that you are more likely to work with a therapist who meets your needs and style.

What Exactly Is Psychotherapy?

Psychotherapy is a fancy word for talk therapy. It is a way to get your mind healthy. Some therapy happens over a very short period, and some can last for years. But even if you begin working with a therapist and continue to do so for a long time, the benefits of talk therapy become apparent quickly for most patients. This is key for women suffering from postpartum problems. It isn't about suddenly feeling "perfect," but about moving closer to a state of happiness or peacefulness. Psychotherapy can help you gain a deeper understanding of yourself and make positive changes. Most psychotherapy tends to be interactive and conversational.

Is Psychotherapy Like Venting to a Friend?

Good therapy should not just be about blowing off steam, though that may be a satisfying by-product. You should feel that you can trust and confide in your therapist as you would a close friend, but therapy is not simply venting. Your therapist is trained to guide you through your problems, rather than simply listen to you talk. By working hard and in a committed way, you can develop insight and awareness about yourself in therapy. Important internal and behavioral changes happen. Chapter 4 discussed some thinking patterns that can prolong your depression. Of course, you can start addressing these on your own, but your therapist can also add a professional perspective to help you understand your thought patterns and how they are affecting you and making you more anxious or depressed.

When you think about the stresses of being a new mom, there are probably a few recurrent themes. Perhaps some have to do with your parents or your partner, with your body, going back to work, or your baby's well-being. Psychotherapy aims to help you have a deeper understanding of your stressors, how they are affecting you, and how you are responding to them so that you can take control of your emotional life regarding these key issues.

Your therapist will listen to you carefully and without judgment. She or he will offer you guidance, and can give you another perspective on things. Most importantly, your therapist will help you move toward change that will make you feel healthier and return to yourself.

How Can Just Talking Make Me Feel Better?

Believe it or not, psychotherapy can change your biology and psychology to help you improve. Cutting-edge research shows that psychotherapy actually leads to real changes in the brain on a biological level, in areas that medication does not target. The learning that happens in psychotherapy creates and strengthens connections between different areas of the brain and changes brain activity to help you feel happier.

> Psychotherapy leads to biological changes in the brain.

Not only will you be able to address the things that are bothering you when you are in therapy, but having a connected and trusting relationship with your therapist can be therapeutic in and of itself. Feeling valued and supported by your therapist goes a long way to helping you recover. You should feel that you are taken seriously and have confidence that your therapist will guide you in the right direction.

How to Get the Most Out of Therapy

1. Take the first step

Get the ball rolling by calling your family doctor to get more information about good therapists near you or by calling someone recommended by a friend who had PPD or PPA. Review the list in Chapter 5 about how to find a mental health professional and check out the Resources section at the back of the book for more information. Just making an appointment can give you a sense of relief and the feeling that you do not have to deal with this alone.

2. Find someone you like and feel comfortable with.

This is such an important aspect. When you are developing a therapeutic relationship with someone, it is essential to feel supported
by this person and to trust him or her. You need to feel like you
are in this process with the right therapist. Along the therapeutic
journey, you may have some sessions that feel like a waste of time
or you may get upset about something your therapist says or does.
The best way to deal with this is to be open and honest with your
therapist. Let her or him know how you feel, which will give both
of you the opportunity to address the problem or concern. Addressing your concerns helps the therapeutic process work for you.
That way, you and your therapist can make necessary changes to
the treatment and your therapist will get a better understanding
of what you really need. Your therapist may be an excellent professional, but she or he can also make mistakes or have "off" days or
say something that strikes a particular nerve for you. The key is
to address this, learn from it, and forge ahead.

If you feel that you are not getting better or that the therapy
does not feel right for you, then you need to let your therapist
know this too. Again, it is best to have an open and frank discussion about your concerns with your therapist, rather than
simply stopping your sessions. If your current therapy is not
the right treatment for you, then your therapist may be able to
steer you in a more suitable direction.

3. Make a real commitment to therapy.

Because therapy requires time and emotional commitment from
you, you need to decide how much you can devote to this. Once
you decide, stay committed to that goal. As with most things,
the more committed you are, the better the outcome will be.
You need to attend your sessions and do what your therapist
asks you to follow up with between sessions.

If you feel unsure, you might want to commit to short-term therapy at first, or even to just a few sessions, and see how that goes. You may find that you benefit from the sessions and want to continue the process. Giving therapy a wholehearted try is a necessary step in getting the most out of it.

4. Make sure you see progress.

When you are suffering from PPD or PPA, you need to feel better *quickly*. You should see some progress within a few weeks of starting treatment. To achieve this, the focus of psychotherapy initially should be in the *here and now* (even if that means addressing how the past may be affecting you here and now). You need to get out of crisis mode and feel better, so you can care for yourself and develop a strong and loving bond with your baby. Of course, issues from your past and deeper problems can emerge in therapy, but it may be best to shelve these at first and address them once you are feeling better. When you have a clearer and more peaceful mind, exploring these other issues in depth can be very beneficial and ward off future episodes of PPD and PPA. For now, pay close attention to how you are feeling and make sure your therapy is helping you recover.

5. Find therapy that suits your budget.

Therapy can be costly, but you can also often find less expensive or free options.

In Canada, if you see a family doctor or a psychiatrist who can provide psychotherapy, you will not have to pay out of pocket because MDs who are also therapists are covered by your provincial health care system. If you cannot find an MD psychotherapist, ask your employer about your benefit package. Many employers offer benefits that include several visits to a therapist, usually a social worker or psychologist. In the US, you can ask your health insurance provider how many therapy sessions are covered under your plan. Your local university or college may also have therapy training programs where students who are learning to be therapists offer a more affordable rate.

Types of Psychotherapy

The best way to find the right type of therapy for you is to have a basic understanding the major kinds of individual and multi-person therapies. These have all been proven to work—but one or two of them may be better suited to your needs.

Let's look at the various forms of individual psychotherapy so you can make an informed choice about your treatment.

Often therapists are familiar with all these types of therapy and use a blend of techniques. If you find that the first kind of therapy or therapist you choose does not feel right, feel free to experiment with different therapists and different types of therapy. What type of therapy you choose does not matter as long as it helps you recover from PPD or PPA and embrace motherhood wholeheartedly.

Psychodynamic

In psychodynamic therapy, you will be encouraged to explore early childhood experiences and relationships and to examine how these impact your problems with PPD or PPA.

There are various types of psychodynamic therapies. Short-term therapies usually last three to four months, with weekly one-hour meetings that are often structured to address specific issues and crises. This type of brief therapy may be great for you if issues from your childhood or with your parents are aggravating your PPD or PPA. You can focus on these underlying problems and develop insight that will help you make changes rapidly.

Long-term psychodynamic therapy is often open-ended, less structured, and can continue for years. People often confuse the terms "psychoanalysis" and "psychotherapy." Psychoanalysis is a form of intense, long-term psychotherapy. This is the therapy Sigmund Freud developed in which the patient is usually lying down, facing away from the therapist. The patient free associates and talks about his or her feelings and experiences. The patient and therapist meet frequently, often up to five days each week, for many years.

Once you feel better, you may want to begin long-term therapy to grapple with issues that have been plaguing you for some time, such as personality quirks or relationship stumbling blocks that tend to recur for you. You can also begin open-ended therapy while you have PPD or PPA, and make headway toward recovery.

Cognitive Behavioral Therapy (CBT)

As mentioned previously, the goals of CBT are to address your distorted thinking and problematic reactions in order to improve your mood and anxiety levels. Hopefully you are already practising some of the CBT skills discussed in Chapter 4. CBT is a short-term therapy that lasts about three to four months. A CBT therapist will ask you to record your thoughts, feelings, behaviors, and symptoms that are triggered in specific situations. In a session, you might review your findings and talk about how to react to a situation with less sadness, self-loathing, or anxiety. CBT can be great for depression and anxiety disorders, including panic disorder, generalized anxiety disorder, obsessive-compulsive disorder, and social phobia.

CBT may be good for you if you do not feel the need to delve into earlier issues, but want to focus on stopping certain reactions, such as panic attacks or specific symptoms that are getting you down.

Interpersonal Psychotherapy (IPT)

IPT is another short-term, focused therapy that continues for three to four months with weekly sessions. IPT is based on the theory that depression emerges when our important relationships change, are stressed, or are lost. For many women with PPD, the focus of IPT is dealing with the transition to motherhood, and how this triggers depression. In IPT you would look at what it means to become a mother; your fantasy about motherhood compared to the reality; what you have given up; which changes are welcomed; and which changes feel too overwhelming. Your IPT therapist will help you understand how this transition has made you depressed and will help you implement changes, including getting better supports, so you will feel better. The ultimate goal of IPT is to treat your depression so you can embrace this new stage in life.

You may want to consider IPT if you believe that your depression results from this life-stage change or from other relationship stressors or losses that occurred at the same time that you became a mother.

IPT is great for PPD and has also been proven to be an effective treatment for bipolar disorder as well as for bulimia nervosa.

As you see, there are different types of individual therapy to meet your current needs and personality. Now you know that you don't have to review your childhood if it isn't what you think you need, that therapy can have a specific time frame and be goal-oriented, and that psychotherapy can also be wide open and last as long as you need, covering any subject that comes up. You can decide which of these is appealing to you and find a therapist to create a suitable plan.

Two's Company and Three or More Is a Group

Individual therapy is often very important for women who have postpartum issues, but sometimes you may need to see a therapist with your partner if relationship issues are looming large. There is much more information about how your partner can be an important part of your recovery in Chapter 9. Group therapy and support groups are other excellent forms of help.

Couples Therapy

Relationship problems that you were able to ignore or deal with on your own before you had a baby have a way of re-emerging when you enter parenthood.

Like Zoe, you may have a partner who went out several nights each week prior to your baby's birth. Before the baby arrived, this did not bother Zoe because she had her own busy social calendar and was happy being at home alone, doing her own thing. But the baby was colicky, difficult to soothe, and slept very little, which drained Zoe's energy. At the same time, Zoe's husband continued to go out regularly and stay out late. Zoe felt that he did not contribute to child care or to much else around the home. However, he felt he was working hard to support his new family and deserved to hang out with his friends because he really needed a break. As Zoe's exhaustion, anger, and resentment increased, she would yell at her partner a lot, which just made him spend more time out of the house. Their relationship deteriorated and Zoe got depressed. They decided to see a couples therapist to address their troubled relationship. After a few sessions, Zoe and her partner learned how to share their needs in a more direct, respectful, and productive way, and Zoe's depression improved.

Sexual issues, financial issues, scheduling issues, sharing the workload and communication issues are all things that couples fight about. It can feel harder to deal with these issues when baby comes along, and this can contribute to PPD. It can be immensely helpful to address these issues in couples therapy. Or, if your relationship has suffered a serious blow since the baby's birth, such as infidelity, a couples therapist can be a neutral third party to help you and your partner talk about difficult issues. Even moderate but very common frustrations, such as who does what around the house and who contributes more to the family, can be part of the issues aggravating postpartum depression and can be discussed in couples therapy.

In couples therapy, you and your partner meet with a therapist to discuss what is troubling you as a couple. As with individual therapy, couples' therapy should first focus on resolving the issues that are contributing to your PPD or PPA. Once you feel better, you and your partner may decide that you need ongoing therapy to discuss other issues.

Although many couples think that if they need to see a therapist this means that the end of their relationship is near, this could not be further from the truth. Couples therapy isn't only for couples planning to break up or who are in seriously destructive or dangerous relationships. It can be immensely helpful for addressing recurring patterns that have been interfering in your communication with your partner. Often minor tweaks to a relationship lead to major benefits. Your relationship will improve and couples therapy will also treat your PPD or PPA.

Group Therapy and Support Groups

Some women love the idea of talking to other moms with similar issues and struggles. Some worry that they will only feel worse after they talk to other moms with PPD because they will take on others' problems. Or, they feel embarrassed and ashamed to reveal their postpartum problems in a more public way. You may think that group therapy is not for you, but it is a wonderful and effective treatment for many women. First, it is one of the best ways to help you realize that you are not alone with your problems. This is a very powerful strength of group therapy. Under the guidance of a professional therapist, group therapy provides the opportunity for you to meet others who understand what you are going through. As well as being supportive of you, other group members can be wonderful sources of inspiration. They will share their own stories of recovery and perhaps you can gain strength and practical ideas from them. Finally, you can address personality issues or behavior patterns that might contribute to your PPD. For example, you can work on addressing issues that keep you isolated from other people. In a group, you will get direct input and feedback from other group members and the therapist, and you can practise new ways of interacting with other people in a safe environment.

Group therapy sessions are led by professional therapists. Some are structured to start and end on a certain date and the same women come each time. More commonly, PPD groups are ongoing and are open to women who come and go, according to their needs. It is great for a mom who has just recently developed PPD or PPA and cannot imagine feeling well to see other women who have been where she is and have made excellent recoveries. If you are considering group therapy as part of your treatment plan, it is often best to combine it with other forms of treatment, such as individual therapy or perhaps medication, which will be discussed in the next chapter. This way, you will continue to process what you learn in the group with your individual therapist or physician, who can also directly monitor your health.

Support groups and self-help groups have similar components to formal group therapy, but are generally not led by a professional therapist. Moms who have recovered from PPD often organize and lead support groups. Some women find this less formal setting easier and less intimidating, while others feel more comfortable in a professionally organized and structured setting. Keep in mind that a support group may not be the right environment for you to work on underlying problems. It is more a place to connect with and learn from other women who have or had PPD or PPA. But the basics of creating a support network, recognizing you are not alone, and sharing wisdom and guidance are all found in good support groups and group therapy.

For some women, going to their group meetings may be their only time to leave the house and socialize each week. Many women, such as Alexandra, tell me that their weekly support group meetings are their "lifeline." Initially, Alexandra admitted to being anxious about attending a support group for new moms with PPD as part of her treatment plan. She always considered herself a private person and was scared that she would be forced to speak about herself in public. However, during the first session when she met the other group members and saw what the support group was about, Alexandra began to feel comfortable. She was assured that everything they talked about was confidential, and she heard from other moms how helpful the group had been in their recovery. During the first few sessions, she listened attentively and was relieved to hear that other women were having similar struggles. She was not alone. After about three sessions, Alexandra was comfortable enough to reveal some things about herself and her struggle with depression as a new mother. When the feedback from the other group members was so supportive and helpful, she really felt understood and validated for the first time. From other group members, Alexandra learned where to find other good resources for her PPD and lots of great baby care information that she had never heard anywhere else. After being in the group for a few months and meeting so many wonderful women who had gone through PPD, Alexandra was no longer depressed and felt that she was ready to "graduate" from her group.

When you are organizing your treatment plan, choose the type of therapy you think best suits your needs and that is available in your area. Feeling comfortable and at ease is essential while you cope with and recover from PPD. Use the resources listed in Chapter 5 and at the end of this book to find a suitable therapist or group near you.

Therapy is an extremely valuable part of a treatment plan for almost any woman experiencing PPD or PPA. However, even the fastest responses to therapy can take several weeks, and some women need immediate care to stop the slide into darker depression and anxiety. In those cases, medication is often helpful and necessary. There are perhaps more myths regarding medications and PPD than any other aspect of treatment, and you probably have your own fears and questions. Medications will be discussed in the next chapter.

Chapter 7
Medications

If you are experiencing PPD or PPA or are concerned that you might, you know by now that you don't need to suffer any longer, because there are safe and effective ways to feel better. You have your at-home arsenal of ideas to try; you are sleeping better and exercising and paying attention to your thoughts. And you have connected with a doctor or therapist. Likely, the topic of medications has come up. For many women medications are the most frightening and controversial aspect of PPD or PPA treatment. Most people share the same worries when it comes to postpartum issues and medication: "What about side effects for me and the baby? How long will I have to take drugs? What about the stigma? Can I still breastfeed? Are these medications addictive? Isn't there any other way?" Good for you for being aware, for asking these and many other questions, and for being concerned and thoughtful about what you put in your body.

For some women, particularly for those with more intense depression or anxiety, taking antidepressant medication can be the best option. Drugs often work extremely well in treating PPD and PPA. This doesn't mean that medication is right or advisable for everyone, and every woman must get the facts and make her own decisions for her particular treatment plan. However, dismissing the option of drugs without gathering the scientific evidence is akin to not seeking treatment because of any one of the myths discussed in the first chapter.

Try to keep an open mind while I explain the commonly used medications for PPD and PPA. I will answer some of the popular questions women have about taking antidepressants, talk about the specific medications for PPD and PPA, and discuss when drugs are and are not appropriate. Then I will tell you about the common side effects and, of course, the latest information about the safety of drugs during breastfeeding. I will also address the issue of dealing with depression if you are pregnant.

Medication is not the answer for everyone who has postpartum emotional concerns. If you have Baby Blues or a few days of overwhelming stress and crying, medication may not be what you need. If you are in a very difficult relationship or have complicated family issues that are impacting how you feel, medication may not be a necessary part of your plan. Your doctor might suggest that you take medication if your symptoms are severe (see the chart on page 65 as a reminder of the degrees of PPD); if you have had a high level of depression or anxiety for a long time; if you have been on antidepressants before and they helped you and were easy for you to take; if you have already made positive changes to your sleep, lifestyle, and support network, but are still feeling really awful. Ultimately, the decision about taking medication is yours and yours alone. Hopefully, the information in this chapter will help you to feel comfortable and well informed.

Medication Myth Busting

Many women are initially reluctant to take medication. Let's address some of the most common misconceptions.

Taking Medication Means I'm Weak

For many people, taking antidepressant medicine feels like a failure. They feel they have not been able to "get it together" by themselves and that "relying" on medicine to feel better is a weakness. (First of all, this self-critical approach may reflect your depressed state of mind, as discussed in Chapter 4.) In fact, taking charge of your health in any way is really a tremendous strength. You have the right to feel good and get better, and to do whatever it takes to help you reach that important goal. If you can recognize that you need help and take steps to feel well, then that is excellent. In the right circumstances, medication can be a key part of your recovery and help you feel stronger and healthier and more like your normal self.

*Medications Confirm That My Problems Are **Real**, and I Want to Forget about This Whole Thing*

Many women find it difficult to acknowledge and admit that they have PPD or PPA. They fear that taking a pill is a strong daily reminder of the situation they are trying to deny or avoid. To get better, you need to first accept that you have an illness and deal with it head-on. It would be wonderful if wishing PPD away would make it disappear, but unfortunately, that is not the case. Developing a good treatment plan that may or may not include medication, and monitoring the plan to see if it is working is the key to recovery. Stay open-minded about your options for treatment and focus on getting better, rather than on wishing the problem away.

If I Need Medication, I Must Really Be Going Crazy

For many people, antidepressants are synonymous with being crazy. While it is true that medication is often needed for more serious forms of PPD or PPA, it only means that you have an illness that needs treatment. Medication can effectively target certain symptoms of PPD or PPA, such as insomnia, poor concentration, confused thinking, energy changes and, of course, depressed mood and very intense worries. Often these symptoms are not easily eliminated with other forms of treatment, and it can be hard to do psychotherapy effectively or to pursue self-help changes when you are dogged by severe symptoms. Like any effective treatment for PPD or PPA, the right medication can help you regain control of your life and help you feel better.

I Want to Try Only Non-medication Treatments

It is reasonable to want to avoid taking medication and to do whatever it takes to get well without taking drugs. Some women feel better about their treatment plan by excluding drugs, practising self-help techniques, making the significant lifestyle changes suggested in Chapter 4, engaging in psychotherapy treatments, and expanding their support network. They find that this plan works for them and helps them feel well. Other women may start out by making these changes and then feel they need something more to truly recover, so they later decide to take medications. And some women will simply find it difficult, if not impossible, to get back on their feet without medicine. Feel free to try what you think might help you through this time. As you are following your treatment plan, pay close attention to your symptoms and how you are feeling. Most importantly, consider changing your treatment plan if you are not getting better or if you are feeling worse after a few weeks. Do what works for you as long as it *really* does work.

I'd Be Too Embarrassed to Tell Anyone That I'm Taking Medication

Unfortunately, this type of thinking is far too common and reflects the stigma of mental illness. By now, you know that PPD is a real illness and sometimes requires a biological treatment: medicine. You would probably not feel ashamed if you had to give yourself insulin injections to manage your diabetes or take antibiotics for your chest infection, so try to think of this as a medical illness that needs to be taken care of. Plus, if you do decide to take medication for PPD or PPA, this is your own business, and no one needs to know about it.

I Can't Breastfeed and Take Medication at the Same Time

You will be surprised to know that there is much good scientific data to show that many medications, including the most commonly prescribed antidepressants, are safe to take when you are breastfeeding. I will discuss this in more detail later in this chapter, but for now, realize that this is a myth based on outdated or false information.

A Fine Balance

Medications are not perfect, of course, and you should be cautious and well informed before making a decision such as this that may have consequences for you, your child, and your family. The decision to take medication or not needs to be taken very seriously. Unfortunately, the effects of depression can also be very damaging to you, your child, and your family. For this reason, you need to weigh the options and reflect on the pros and cons of any specific medication and any treatment decision. The major advantage of a medicine is that it helps you feel better quickly. The cons to think about are any side effects of the medication and, if you are nursing, if exposure to it will affect your baby. Ultimately, you need to feel comfortable with whichever type of treatment you choose, and I will give you the information to help you make a well-informed decision. Please also consider that if you decide not to treat your serious depression or anxiety, this decision will also impact you, your baby, and your family.

Commonly Asked Questions About Taking Medication

Now, let's answer some of the most frequently asked questions about taking medication.

When Will the Drug Start Working?

It usually takes about four to six weeks to feel the maximum benefit of an antidepressant when it is at an effective dose. Some people feel that a drug is very helpful after a few days, while it may take others a few weeks to begin to feel the benefit. You may notice that your energy, sleep, and appetite improve very quickly. It can take longer before you actually start to feel happier. Others may notice that you seem better before you actually sense the improvement yourself, so be sure to ask those close to you for feedback on how they think you are doing.

After you are prescribed a medication, your doctor should monitor you closely to see how you respond to the drug, to see if you have any serious side effects, and to answer any questions you may have about the treatment. When you begin taking a medication, you should see your doctor regularly to check if the dose needs to be altered. Often it is best to start on a low dose and then slowly increase it if necessary. Each time you see your doctor, she or he will ask if there is any improvement. If there is no change, and you are comfortable taking a higher dose, then the dose may be increased. This should continue until you and your physician feel that the drug and the dose are working well for you. The key is to see and feel improvement within days to weeks.

If you have severe postpartum depression or anxiety that is preventing you from functioning and caring for yourself and your baby, it may be hard to wait four to six weeks until the medication is effective. Please let your doctor know how you are doing every step of the way and make sure you have supportive and caring people to help you through this time. You need to be safe and your baby needs to be well cared for.

Here are a few tips to remember when you are taking an antidepressant:

1. The first drug that you try may not be the right one for you, but don't give up hope.
Sometimes it takes time, patience, and trial and error to find a medication that is right for you. People often have idiosyncratic reactions or unexpected side effects from a medication. Since there are several antidepressants that you can try, don't despair if the first one you are prescribed is not the right one for you.

2. More than one drug may be needed.
If you do not feel any benefits from a decent dose of medication after four to six weeks, there are a few options. First, you may need an even higher dose of the drug for another few weeks. Next, your doctor may switch you to another antidepressant. Sometimes, if you have partially benefited from an antide-pressant drug you are taking and you are on a high dose, your physician may suggest adding another medication to your regimen. You are not a "lost cause" if one antidepressant cannot get your symptoms under control. Often patients who are very depressed require more than one antidepressant medication to feel better.

3. Your medication regimen may need fine-tuning to deal with side effects.

You may find that the drug you are taking makes you feel drowsy and all you want to do is sleep. This does not mean that this drug is not for you. There could be an easy solution to your problem. By taking the drug in the evening, you may sleep well at night and feel more energetic during the day. Alternatively, if you feel a bit hyper from your antidepressant, you can take it in the morning so that you can benefit from the extra energy and sleep better at night. I will discuss side effects in detail later.

How Long Will I Have to Take These Drugs?

The answer to this question depends on the severity of your depression, and how many previous episodes of depression you have had.

If you have a very severe episode, it may take longer to get your symptoms under control. For an episode of depression to be considered fully treated or in full remission, you need to feel well for at least six months. Expert consensus is that you stay on an antidepressant, at the same dose that helped get you well, for six to 12 months after you are feeling well. (It may take a few weeks or months to get you on the right medication and the right dose before you begin feeling healthy, so start counting only once you are well. Don't start counting from the time you take the first tablet.) It is not recommended to stop taking your drugs before the six-month mark because the symptoms of depression and anxiety are likely to return if you stop your medication too soon.

If you want to stop taking your medication, and you have had only one or two depressive episodes, you may do so after six to 12 months of wellness. However, often it is best to stay on a drug for at least one year to prevent a relapse of your symptoms. If you want to stop taking your medication, but the timing coincides with a potentially stressful life event, such as going back to work, weaning the baby off breastfeeding, moving, or the winter holidays, it may be best to wait until there is less external stress in your life to give yourself the best chance for staying well.

If you have a history of severe depressive episodes that have been hard to treat, or more than three depressive episodes in the past, or more than two episodes in the past five years, or a long history of anxiety, the six-month to 1-year mark for stopping your medication may not apply to you. You should stay on your medication for at least two years and perhaps longer, in order to stay well and prevent a relapse. Take one step at a time, and stay in open communication with your doctor.

How Do I Come off Antidepressants?

When you are feeling well and would like to stop your medication, be sure to consult with your doctor. You should slowly taper off your antidepressant over a period of several weeks. If you stop your medication abruptly, you may experience unpleasant symptoms or a "discontinuation syndrome." About 20 percent of people on antidepressants experience unpleasant withdrawal symptoms if they stop taking them suddenly. These include flu-like symptoms, difficulty sleeping, anxiety, agitation, nausea, dizziness, and sometimes electric-shock like sensations. Although they are certainly unpleasant, these symptoms are usually manageable and last one to two weeks. Discontinuation syndromes can be particularly severe when discontinuing paroxetine (Paxil) or venlafaxine (Effexor) because these drugs leave your body quickly. Fluoxetine (Prozac) is not usually associated with discontinuation symptoms because it takes a long time to leave your body.

The best way to deal with a discontinuation syndrome is by preventing it from happening. You and your doctor can devise a plan to taper off your medication gradually. You can reduce the dose of your drug by a small amount every week.

Before you even consider stopping your antidepressant, be sure that your depression or anxiety is fully treated. Once you stop the drug, it is wise to continue to follow up with your physician for a while to make sure that your illness does not return.

Are Antidepressant Medications Addictive?

This is a very common fear and misconception. People often think antidepressants are addictive because they feel awful when they stop taking their pills suddenly, but antidepressants are *not* considered addictive substances since they are not the types of drugs that will make you feel high and leave you craving more. If you feel badly when you stop your medication, it usually means that you have a discontinuation syndrome (as described above) or your symptoms of depression and anxiety have not fully resolved or they have returned. It may be too soon to stop the medicine or you may have to taper off more slowly.

Will Medication Change My Personality or Make Me Feel High or Numb?

Your personality consists of stable characteristics that don't change over time and won't fluctuate when you are on medication. Antidepressant medication will not change who you are or your identity and will not make you feel like you are high. Some women notice that they feel a bit flat when they take antidepressants. They find that they don't cry easily and do not feel as sad and that they also have a harder time feeling very happy. Usually women who are used to having extreme ups and downs as part of their illness experience this. It may be that with medication, your moods remain in a more normal range and don't fluctuate as intensely as they did before treatment. Most of the time, new moms are relieved that the medication helps prevent them from feeling the intense sadness and worries that they felt before. Your personality will not undergo a dramatic change while you are taking antidepressants, but the medicine will help you return to the real you.

If you do feel "out of it," then you may not be on the right medication or the right dose. Please discuss this with your doctor so that you can improve your treatment.

Some women with PPD or PPA may be taking medication for the first time for an underlying depression or anxiety that they have had for years, and they finally feel well. It feels so different from the intense worry, irritability, and sadness they are used to.

Am I at Increased Risk of Suicide If I Take Antidepressants?
Recently there has been a lot of controversy about the relationship between antidepressant medications and suicide. Of course, this is frightening for the millions of people who take antidepressants every day. Much of the concern about suicide has centered on children and adolescents who take antidepressants. This has led the US FDA and Health Canada to put warnings on these drugs. Similar advisories have been issued in the UK. However, it is important to emphasize that the research on risks for children and adolescents showed an increase in suicidal thinking, but not in completed suicides. Some people suggest that this finding reflects an increased likelihood that suicidal thoughts are mentioned to the doctor as opposed to an actual increase in the thoughts themselves. Suicidal thinking and completed suicide events are two very

different things. (Of course, the thoughts often precede the act and need to be taken seriously.) At the same time that antidepressant prescription rates have increased, suicide rates among young people have actually decreased. A recent study showed that when antidepressant prescriptions were decreased, rates of completed suicides increased.

In reality, people who are depressed often have suicidal thinking as a symptom of their depression. Sometimes when an antidepressant starts working, your energy and thinking improve before your mood gets better, as previously discussed. At this time, although it is extremely rare, people who are very suicidal may have the wherewithal to act on their suicidal thinking, which may have not yet subsided, whereas before they began taking medication, they were too depressed to act on these thoughts. It is important to stay in close and constant contact with your doctor when you have very bad PPD and are starting treatment. Perhaps you should see your doctor weekly for the first several weeks of treatment to monitor the efficacy of the medication and any suicidal thoughts. Once the treatment seems to be helping and your side effects are under control, you may be able to visit your doctor every two weeks for a few months, and then less frequently as you get stronger and healthier.

Is This Doctor Right for Me?

It is important that you have a good, honest, and open relationship with your doctor, as previously discussed. This means that you need to feel helped, that you trust your doctor, and that you are both working toward the same goals.

Your doctor should be able to give you details about the treatment you are receiving, and about the side effects of treatment as well as its risks and benefits. You need to feel comfortable asking questions, telling your physician if you have doubts about the treatment, or letting him or her know if you have troubling side effects.

If you decide not to fill the prescription or take the drugs that you discussed with your doctor, please be honest about this with him or her. It is better to talk about this than to stop treatment without consulting your physician.

Whenever you decide that you want to stop medication, discuss this with your doctor. I know the temptation is to stop taking prescribed drugs if you feel they are not helping you or are causing too many side effects. You may be worried about how your doctor will react to this and avoid him or her. Or, if you feel angry toward your physician, the temptation is to cancel the next appointment or not show up at all and never see your doctor again. But for the sake of your health and well-being and that of your family, please follow through with your doctor.

If you feel that your current health care provider is un-satisfactory, you have a few options. Either you can return to see him or her to be guided in the right direction, or request a referral to another health care professional, or you can ask around to find someone who is right for you. Again, you may be most comfortable with someone who specializes in helping women with postpartum problems, if this is available in your area. There is a list of specialized programs in the Resources section at the back of the book. Be sure to keep the momentum going to find someone who can be helpful and supportive in a way that feels right for you.

Which Medication Is the Right One for Me?

Once you and your doctor decide that you will take medication, there are several things you should share with your doctor to determine the right drug for you. There are many different safe and effective options and the final decision will be determined by the factors discussed below.

1. Tell your doctor if you have ever had depression or anxiety or another psychiatric issue before, and if you took medication in the past. Let your doctor know if the previous drug controlled your symptoms and about any significant side effects. If the medicine you took in the past is considered safe for breastfeeding (if you are nursing), then this is usually the place to start. If something worked before, then use it again. Conversely, if your doctor suggests a medication that you did not like before, avoid this option.

2. Remember to mention any physical problems you have had or any other drugs you are currently taking. Obviously, if certain antidepressants worsen your medical condition or cannot be taken with other medications you need to take, you should avoid these drugs.

3. Discuss the symptoms that are most troublesome to you right now. Some drugs are particularly good at targeting certain symptoms, so you can select the right medication for your particular symptoms. For example, if you are very anxious, you can avoid taking a drug that will heighten your anxiety.

4. If you know that you want to avoid certain side effects, such as sexual side effects, you and your physician may choose one drug over another.

5. Medications that any close family members have taken are important to mention. If there is a drug that worked well for your close blood relatives, then this will likely be a good choice for you too.

6. Consider ahead of time how much you can spend on medication each month so that you and your doctor can find drugs that are within your budget.

Generally, most women who have PPD or PPA and who have never been prescribed an antidepressant start with a selective serotonin reuptake inhibitor (SSRI) or a selective serotonin/norepinephrine reuptake inhibitor (SNRI). (Although they are called antidepressants, both classes of drugs are commonly used to treat anxiety disorders as well.) There is detailed information about these medications in the next section.

Which Medications Are Used to Treat PPD and PPA?

The medications that are commonly used to treat PPD and PPA work very well. Between 70 percent and 80 percent of people feel much better when they take antidepressants. PPD and PPA respond just as well to antidepressants as other forms of depression and anxiety do. In fact, the vast majority of women with PPD and PPA respond well to medication and usually feel much better quickly. Since there is no single drug that is recommended above all others for PPD and PPA, and no single choice that is right for every woman, I will discuss various antidepressants and focus on the medications that are the most effective and most commonly prescribed for PPD or PPA. I have created a chart (p.169-71) you can refer to for an overview of the antidepressant drugs, particularly the newer medications. I will also explain the most frequent side effects associated with antidepressants and how to address these issues if they occur. (When the brand name of the drug is different in Canada, the United States and the UK, the name of the drug in each country will be given in parentheses. Otherwise, please assume the name is the same.)

There are many good options available to suit your personal needs. The medications listed below are by no means the only ones that may be helpful for you. There are many drugs available, and new ones are always coming onto the market. However, this section is meant to be a guide to help you decide how to begin or how to proceed.

Antidepressants

Most women with PPD or PPA who take medication will usually start with an antidepressant drug.

How Do Antidepressants Work?

As discussed earlier, depression or anxiety emerges when there is an imbalance of important brain chemicals, including serotonin and norepinephrine and sometimes dopamine. Antidepressants help you feel better because they rebalance your brain chemicals to normal levels. Different medications target different chemicals.

Selective Serotonin Reuptake Inhibitors (SSRIs)

Selective serotonin reuptake inhibitors are the most commonly prescribed class of antidepressants for PPD and depression in general. They have been around since the late 1980s, and target the brain chemical serotonin, which regulates your mood and anxiety level. Too little serotonin is thought to result in depression and anxiety. These drugs enable more serotonin to bathe the brain in places where it needs to be. The drugs do not create serotonin, but they prevent it from being taken away from key brain regions. The medications in this class are: sertraline (Zoloft, UK: Lustral), paroxetine (Paxil, UK: Seroxat), fluoxetine (Prozac), fluvoxamine (Luvox, UK: Faverin), citalopram (Celexa, UK: Cipramil), escitalopram (Canada & UK: Cipralex, US: Lexapro).

Other New Antidepressants

Venlafaxine (Effexor, UK: Efexor) and duloxetine (Cymbalta) are in the class of drugs called selective serotonin/norepinephrine reuptake inhibitors (SNRIs). These medications act on two main brain chemicals or neurotransmitters, serotonin and norepinephrine. Venlafaxine may become more effective as the dose is increased because it also acts on the brain chemical dopamine at high doses.

Bupropion (Wellbutrin) is an antidepressant that acts on norepinephrine and dopamine. It is good for depression and ADHD, but may not be as good for anxiety disorders.

Mirtazapine (US & Canada: Remeron, UK: Zispin) is an antidepressant that works on norepinephrine and serotonin and works well for depression and anxiety. It is often helpful for treating insomnia related to PPD.

Tricyclic Antidepressants (TCAs)

Tricyclics, which are good drugs for depression and anxiety, have been in use since the 1950s and were commonly used until SSRIs entered the market. Most TCAs work primarily on norepinephrine, but they also affect serotonin and dopamine. These drugs are as effective as SSRIs, but have become less popular because of their many side effects (weight gain, constipation, sedation, dry mouth, blurred vision, low blood pressure, and urinary retention) and the danger they pose if taken as an overdose. They are also unsafe for women with certain heart problems. TCAs are not commonly prescribed today unless the newer antidepressants have been tried and found to be ineffective.

Drugs in this class include: amitriptyline (Elavil, UK: Tryp-tizol), clomipramine (Anafranil), desipramine (Norpramin), imipramine (Tofranil), nortriptylene (Canada: Aventyl, US: Pamelor, UK: Allegron), and doxepin (Sinequan). Of the TCAs, nortriptylene has been researched the most for use during breastfeeding and is considered safe. Doxepin, on the other hand, should be avoided by nursing moms.

Monoamine Oxidase Inhibitors (MAOIs)
Monoamine oxidase inhibitors is an older class of antidepres-sants that work on serotonin, norepinephrine, and dopamine. Although these are very effective antidepressants and anti-anxi-ety drugs, they are rarely prescribed unless absolutely necessary because they can have very dangerous interactions with certain types of medications and food. Tyramine-containing foods—such as aged and fermented cheeses, smoked meats, fava beans, soy products, and some beers—should be avoided when taking MAOIs. MAOIs are not commonly used by women with PPD and there is limited data about safety during breastfeeding. For these reasons, and because of the dietary and drug limitations required with MAOIs, they are reserved for women who do not improve with other medications.

The drugs in this class include phenelzine (Nardil), tranylcy-promine (Parnate), and isocarboxazid (Marplan) in the US.

Side Effects of Antidepressants
One of the main reasons many women are reluctant to take an antidepressant is they are concerned about possible side effects. Unfortunately, almost every drug has some type of side effect. Some side effects are minimal, not too bothersome, and go away soon after treatment begins, while other side effects may be intolerable and may linger. It is impossible to know in

advance exactly how you will respond to a given drug and which side effects, if any, you will experience. Fortunately, many side effects do go away on their own and there are ways to manage and minimize other side effects.

Troubling side effects (and not knowing how to manage them) is one of the main reasons why people stop taking their medicines. While you need to be aware of how a drug is affecting you and monitor this closely, please do not let your worries about potential side effects deter you from trying an antidepressant if you really need it or stop you from taking it if you are on it. Often, if you can tolerate a few days to a few weeks of unpleasant side effects, they will subside and the drug will start working for you. Again, I know this is easier said than done, but being patient really can and does pay.

In this section, I will cover the most common side effects associated with antidepressants and provide suggestions about how you or your doctor can handle them. Remember that not all of these will happen to you and you may not have any side effects at all, but it is important to be aware of the various side effects so that you will know how to deal with them. Some of the suggestions listed here are things that you can do on your own to help ease the side effects. You will need to speak to your prescribing physician to add new medication or to make changes to your current medicine. In the meantime, please write down any side effects you have, if you start taking a new drug, and tell your doctor. And be sure to tell your doctor immediately if you feel much worse when you start a medication.

Jitteriness/agitation

- Is common when starting antidepressants, especially SSRIs or SNRIs, but often goes away after a few days
- Can be a symptom of depression and anxiety, but if it gets

worse when you start a medication, tell your doctor
- May need to reduce your dose or increase the dose on a slower schedule
- May need to add calming medication, such as a benzodiazepine

Headache
- May begin when starting medication, but often goes away after one to two weeks
- Take acetaminophen (Tylenol), paracetamol in the UK or ibuprofen (Advil)

Nausea and reduced appetite
- May begin when starting medication, and often goes away after one to two weeks
- Take antidepressant with meals
- Take dimenhydrinate (Canada: Gravol, US: Dramamine) as needed
- Switch to controlled-release (CR) or extended-release (XR) formulations of your medicine, if available
- May need to lower your dose or switch to another antidepressant
- Choose foods that are bland and easy on your stomach, such as crackers or bananas

Dry mouth
- May be continuous, but can improve with time
- Chew sugarless gum or suck on sugarless candy
- Drink lots of water

Loose bowels or diarrhea
- Is more common with SSRIs and SNRIs
- Often goes away after a few days

- May need to lower your dose
- Drink plenty of water to stay hydrated

Constipation
- Is more common with TCAs and bupropion, and may be continuous
- Increase your fiber intake by eating more bran, whole grains, fruits, and vegetables
- Drink more water
- Consider taking a stool softener or a laxative

Fatigue and lethargy
- Take your medicine at bedtime
- Switch to a less sedating drug, such as bupropion
- Don't drive or operate machinery until this side effect diminishes
- If you are fatigued during the day because you are not sleeping at night, ask your doctor about prescribing a sleep medication until your body adjusts to the antidepressant
- May also be a symptom of depression, but if it gets worse on the medication, tell your doctor

Insomnia
- Is worse with SSRIs and bupropion
- Can be a symptom of PPD or PPA as well as a side effect; note if it gets worse when you start an antidepressant
- Take your medication in the morning
- May need to lower your dose
- Avoid caffeine, especially in the afternoon and evening, and avoid exercising later in the day
- Avoid napping late in the day
- Ask your doctor about prescribing a sleep medication

until your body adjusts to the medication and your
depression or anxiety improves

Sexual issues
- Reduced libido, difficulty having an orgasm, or less genital
  sensation are the common sexual side effects
- Women with PPD or PPA (and most women who have
  recently had a baby) are often not feeling sexual anyway,
  so using these drugs may not directly impact your sex
  life, and in fact may help you to get better more quickly,
  thereby improving your sex life
- Is worse with SSRIs
- Reducing your dose or taking your pills after you have sex
  (rather than in the hours before) may help to address the
  sexual side effects; be sure to discuss these options with
  your doctor because they may impact your recovery
- Consider switching to another antidepressant, such as
  bupropion or mirtazapine, that is less likely to have sexual
  side effects
- Ask your doctor about adding a small dose of bupropion
  to your current medication
- Discuss using sildenafil (Viagra) with your doctor; it has
  recently been shown to work well for women who have
  sexual side effects from antidepressants

Weight gain
- Is worse with mirtazapine, TCAs, and MAOIs, but may
  also affect 18 percent of people who take SSRIs for more
  than six months
- Eat healthy, well-balanced meals and exercise
- Meet with a nutritionist
- Consider switching to another antidepressant, such as
  bupropion, that will not cause weight gain

Drug Name *	Drug Class	Dose Range**	General Symptoms Targeted	Notable Side Effects***	Peaks in Milk (hours)	Safety While Breastfeeding ****	Safety for Pregnancy	Notes
Antidepressants:								
Sertraline	SSRI	50–200 mg	Depression and anxiety	May have least amount of weight gain among SSRIs	6	Yes, is considered one of safest drugs for nursing	Appears safe	Good first choice for nursing moms
Paroxetine	SSRI	10–60 mg	Depression and anxiety	May have most amount of weight gain among SSRIs	5	Yes, is considered one of safest drugs for nursing	Recent controversies about cardiac defects but it appears safe.	Good first choice for nursing moms
Fluoxetine	SSRI	20–80 mg	Depression and anxiety	—	6-8	Yes, but may have higher levels than other SSRIs	Has most safety data of all SSRIs	Good choice for pregnancy
Citalopram	SSRI	10–60mg	Depression and anxiety	—	4-5	Yes, but may have higher levels than other SSRIs	Appears safe	—

Drug Name *	Drug Class	Dose Range**	General Symptoms Targeted	Notable Side Effects***	Peaks in Milk (hours)	Safety While Breastfeeding ****	Safety for Pregnancy	Notes
Fluvoxamine (Luvox)	SSRI	50–300 mg	Depression and anxiety	—	1.5–8	Limited info, but it seems safe	Appears safe	—
Escitalopram	SSRI	10–20 mg	Depression and anxiety	—	—	No published data available.	Limited data	—
Venlafaxine	SNRI	75–300 mg	Depression and anxiety	High blood pressure at higher doses	Standard: 2 Sustained Release (SR): 5–6	Appears safe	Appears safe	—
Duloxetine	SNRI	60–120 mg	Depression and anxiety	—	6	—	—	—
Bupropion	Norepinephrine and dopamine	Standard: 225–450 mg Sustained Release (SR): 150–300 mg	Depression, ADHD	May cause seizures if dose is increased quickly or if any single dose is greater than 150 mg or total dose is greater than 450 mg	1–2	Low levels in milk, but case report of seizure in exposed six-month-old	Limited data, but appears safe	Does *not* have sexual and cardiac side effects, no weight gain, may increase anxiety, not recommended if someone is bulimic
Mirtazapine	Norepinephrine, and serotonin	15–45 mg	Depression, anxiety, and insomnia	Significant weight gain and fatigue; less likely to cause stomach upset	2	Limited data, but appears safe	Limited data	Not a lot of data re: nursing and PPD
Nortriptylene	Tricyclic (TCA)	40–200 mg	Depression and anxiety	Weight gain, constipation, dry mouth, low blood pressure, urinary retention, blurred vision	2–6	Yes, is considered one of safest antidepressants for nursing	Appears safe	Older drug with more side effects; not likely first choice

Amitriptylene	TCA	75–300 mg	Depression and anxiety	Weight gain, constipation, dry mouth, low blood pressure, urinary retention, blurred vision	2–8	Yes, safe	Appears safe	Older drug with more side effects; not likely first choice
Phenelzine	MAOI	15–90 mg	Anxiety and depression that have not responded to other medication	Very dangerous: high blood pressure if tyramine-free diet is not followed	1.5–4	Limited data	Limited data	Not first choice due to food restrictions
Tranylcypromine	MAOI	30–60 mg	Anxiety and depression that have not responded to other medication	Very dangerous: high blood pressure if tyramine-free diet is not followed	2.5–4	Limited data	Limited data	Not first choice due to food restrictions

* I have used the generic names in this chart and noted the brand names earlier in the chapter.

** The dose ranges listed are the official ranges for each of the drugs, but your doctor may, under certain circumstances, put you on a higher or lower dose.

*** Safety while breastfeeding is defined as the baby getting less than 10 percent of the maternal dose.

**** For a full list of side effects, see the section on side effects. This section highlights significant side effects of a drug, if applicable.

Other Medications That May Be Needed

Sometimes other types of drugs are needed instead of an anti-depressant and often other types are added to an antidepressant, for a short time.

Antianxiety Medication

As you can see in the chart, many of the drugs used as anti-depressants, including SSRIs, SNRIs, mirtazapine, and TCAs, are also effective treatments for anxiety. These are the best long-term treatments for anxiety symptoms and disorders, but they sometimes take several weeks to work. Sometimes anxiety is so severe and debilitating that you need immediate relief. If this is the case, you may be prescribed a drug called a benzodiazepine. Benzodiazepines, or "benzos," help you relax and feel calmer immediately. They are often prescribed to treat anxiety, to help deal with the agitation that is sometimes a side effect when starting antidepressants, and to treat insomnia. They can be taken at the same time as antidepressants. Benzodiazepines are meant to be used as a short-term treatment. Diazepam (Valium), clonazepam (Canada & UK: Rivotril, US: Klonopin), lorazepam(Ativan), and alprazolam (Xanax) are commonly used benzodiazepines.

The main side effects from benzodiazepines are drowsiness and daytime tiredness. By taking the lowest possible dose that is still helpful, you can minimize this side effect.

Many women are afraid of becoming addicted to benzo-diazepines. However, when they are taken at very low doses for a few weeks to help you feel calmer or to sleep, you are *very* unlikely to get addicted. (Most women with PPD or PPA require only low doses.) If they are being used for anxiety when starting an antidepressant, they can be stopped once your body has adjusted to the antidepressant and the antidepressant has kicked in. I have never seen any woman treated for PPD or PPA develop an addiction to benzodiazepines if she has not already had another substance-abuse problem. Women usually want to discontinue these medications quickly once their troubling symptoms are under control, and they usually have no trouble tapering off and stopping these medications within a few weeks or months.

Benzodiazepines should not be stopped abruptly. Instead, you should taper off slowly under your doctor's supervision. By gradually reducing your dose, you will avoid any withdrawal symptoms, which include anxiety, agitation, and insomnia. Also, if you stop the medication prematurely, there is a risk that your initial bothersome symptoms will recur.

Benzodiazepines are considered safe for breastfeeding mothers because they enter the breast milk at less than 5 percent of the concentration in the mother's body. Lorazepam is preferable for nursing mothers because lower levels of this drug accumulate in the breast milk and it stays in your body for less time. It is also good to know that lorazepam will be in your body for one to six hours after you take it, so you can nurse after the six-hour mark without exposing your baby to much of the drug. Regardless of the benzodiazepine that you are prescribed, if you are nursing, you should monitor your baby for signs of extreme drowsiness or difficulty breastfeeding.

Sleep Medication

The benzodiazepines are also frequently prescribed to treat sleep problems for new mothers.

Zopiclone (Canada: Imovane, UK: Zimovane) is a sleeping pill commonly prescribed as a short-term treatment or for occasional use for insomnia. Once taken, it will help you fall asleep and stay asleep for about six to eight hours, depending on the dose. It is safe to take in combination with antidepressants. Zopiclone is considered safe during breastfeeding as only 1.4 percent of the mother's dose enters the baby's body.

The main side effects of zopiclone are daytime sleepiness and a bitter taste. Zopiclone is not considered addictive unlike the benzodiazepines as it is a different chemical. Zopiclone can be used as needed for a few weeks or months. When you stop taking it, you may find that it takes a few nights until you can fall asleep easily again. You should not have withdrawal symptoms when you stop taking it.

In the United States and UK, zolpidem (US: Ambien, UK: Stilnoct), zaleplon (Sonata), and eszopiclone (Lunesta: US only) are commonly prescribed sleeping medications that are similar to zopiclone. Zolpidem is considered safe for breast-feeding moms, and although there is less direct information about zaleplon and eszopiclone, these are also considered safe while breastfeeding.

Trazodone (Desyrel, UK: Molipaxin) was originally used as an antidepressant. It is now often used in lower doses as a sleeping pill because it is quite sedating. It may be used while breastfeeding.

Antipsychotic Medication
If postpartum depression or anxiety is very severe, or if a woman has postpartum psychosis or bipolar disorder, an antipsychotic medication may be required. The most commonly prescribed antipsychotic drugs for women with postpartum problems are olanzapine (Zyprexa), quetiapine (Seroquel), and risperidone (Risperdal). More recently, ziprasidone (Canada: Zeldox, US and UK: Geodon) has become available in Canada as well as the US and UK, and aripiprazole (Abilify) is available in the US and UK. These are all newer medications. Sometimes older antipsychotics, such as haloperidol, are prescribed.

If a woman is taking haloperidol while breastfeeding, less than 3 percent enters the breast milk, so she may breastfeed. Although there is limited data, reports show that less than 5 percent of quetiapine enters the breast milk, so this drug may be compatible with breastfeeding. There is minimal data regarding the other antipsychotic drugs and breastfeeding, but preliminary data indicate that olanzapine and risperidone are also safe. Babies whose mothers are nursing while taking antipsychotic medication should be monitored for drowsiness.

If you require an antipsychotic medication, this indicates that you have a more serious psychiatric illness and will need close and continuous monitoring by your physician.

Medications and Breastfeeding

Can I Breastfeed While Taking Medications?

If you are breastfeeding, the thought of taking medication may make you feel anxious, scared, and ambivalent. On the one hand, you need stronger and quicker relief from depression or anxiety, but you also worry that the medication will be harmful for your baby. The good news is that research over the past few years has shown that most antidepressants are safe to take while breastfeeding. You can take medication and nurse your baby at the same time. (The commonly used drug reference resources, the *Physician's Desk Reference* (PDR) in the US or the *Compendium of Pharmaceuticals and Specialties* (CPS) in Canada have warnings against taking medication while breastfeeding. However, the information in these resources does not reflect the most up-to-date literature on this subject.) Please refer to the medication chart to see the latest safety data about antidepressants and nursing.

According to the American Academy of Pediatrics, a substance is considered safe if it enters the breast milk at less than 10 percent of the dose in the mother's blood. The new antidepressants that have been studied have been found to enter breast milk in very small amounts, which are considered compatible with breastfeeding.

The next question is what happens to the baby when she or he is exposed to low levels of antidepressants via breast milk. It seems that most full-term, healthy babies whose nursing mothers take antidepressants have small or undetectable amounts of the medication in their bloodstream. Even if they ingest some of these drugs through breast milk, healthy babies are able to process and rid them from their bodies. In most studies, there have been no reports of problems associated with babies being exposed to antidepressants through breast milk. The few harmful effects that have been noted are: poor sleep, colic, irritability, difficulty feeding, and drowsiness. More seriously, one baby who was exposed to bupropion reportedly had a seizure. In most of these cases, it was impossible to conclude if it was the drug that caused these problems, or if it was another drug the mother was taking, or if a completely separate issue caused these symptoms. The message from the existing data is that concerns have been reported, most of them are not serious, and they are rather unspecific and difficult to link directly to the medication.

If your baby is very premature or has a serious medical condition, such as a liver problem, that may hinder the way the drug is cleared from his or her system, you need to consult your pediatrician about continuing to nurse while taking an antidepressant.

Because the research about antidepressants and breastfeeding is ongoing, we do not have extensive long-term data about the effects on grown children. It is important to emphasize that what we do know points to the fact that infants exposed to antidepressants via breast milk do not appear to have any long-term damage in terms of mental, cognitive, or physical effects. Expert consensus is that it is safe to breastfeed while taking most antidepressants.

The most well-studied drugs for breastfeeding are nortriptylene, fluoxetine, paroxetine, and sertraline. They have also been on the market for the longest time. Since it seems that fluoxetine accumulates at higher rates in breast milk and in exposed infants, we do not usually start with this drug. We usually start with an SSRI, such as sertraline or paroxetine.

If I Am Already on an Antidepressant That May Be Less Safe While Breastfeeding, Should I Switch to Another Medication?

The question of switching to another medication that may be safer for breastfeeding is a complicated one. It really depends on your history of depression and anxiety and your previous response to medication.

If you have a history of severe, difficult-to-treat depression and are currently taking a drug that is keeping you well, it is not a good idea to switch medications. If you have found a drug and a dose that work for you, it is best to stick with that to prevent a relapse of your depression, particularly since most antidepressants appear to be relatively safe for nursing moms to take. Switching to a new medication that may take time to work or may not work for you is a risky proposition when you are in a vulnerable state and need to be well. Plus, switching would expose your baby to two medications, and there is no information about the effects of being exposed to two drugs.

If you have had one or two mild or moderate episodes of depression that did not require medication or that responded quickly and easily to an antidepressant that has less breastfeeding data, you can try to take a drug that has more research data to back up its use. Because your illness is milder and more easily treatable, the risks of trying something new are much lower. Together with your physician, you need to weigh the pros and cons of any medication you might take.

If you are pregnant and are concerned that the medication you are taking may not be the best one for breastfeeding, it is usually inadvisable to switch drugs. First of all, the baby is exposed to significantly more of the drug *in utero* than she or he would be through breast milk. Second, if you need a medication during pregnancy, you do not want to risk relapse by stopping or changing your drugs when you are vulnerable in the postpartum period. Again, this would expose your baby to a second medication. Later in this chapter I will talk about taking antidepressants during pregnancy.

Can I Do Anything So My Baby Is Exposed to Less Medicine?
New mothers who are nursing often wonder if there are ways to limit the amount of medication in their breast milk. Again the evidence shows that taking most antidepressants is safe, but here are a few suggestions:

1. Take the lowest possible dose that is helpful
The lower the dose of your medication, the less the baby will be exposed to. The goal is to take the lowest level of medication that works for you. Taking a dosage that does not fix your depression is certainly not advisable, so work with your doctor to get your medication to the right level and keep it there.

2. Time your medication
By taking your medication immediately after you nurse your baby, before what you think will be his or her longest sleep period, you may lower the amount of drug the baby gets at the next feeding. Or, see the medication chart to find out when

your medicine will peak in your milk and try to nurse when your drug levels are lower.

3. Pump and dump

Try a "pump and dump" regimen to limit your baby's exposure to an antidepressant. When your medication is at its highest level in your blood, use a breast pump to pump your milk and discard it so that your baby is not exposed to the highest concentrations of the antidepressant. To make this work, you need to find out when your medication is at its maximum peak in your bloodstream (see the medication chart). Many antidepressant drugs will be at their highest concentration in your bloodstream six to eight hours after you take your drug. If there is a large range of time that the drug peaks, it may be trickier to work with this information. This option may be hard if you have a newborn who nurses every two to three hours around the clock, but it can work well for older babies. This regimen works well for sertraline in particular to lower the amount of the medication the baby is exposed to.

4. More pumping

When you know that the medication level in your body is lower, you can pump some breast milk and refrigerate it for later use. Pumping can be difficult and time consuming, but this is an option you can try.

I'm Breastfeeding and Taking Antidepressants, So What Should I Look for in My Baby?

You know your baby better than anyone else. Keep a close eye on your baby for the following signs:

1. extreme lethargy
2. excessive crying, irritability, or fussiness
3. difficulty feeding

Of course, many newborns usually have some of these characteristics, but if you find there is a change in your baby's temperament or habits, please let your doctor know immediately. Trust your mothering instincts on this.

Whether or not you notice any problems in your baby, please inform your pediatrician or family physician if you are taking an antidepressant (or any other medication) so she or he can monitor the baby for any potential problems or side effects. Routine monitoring of your baby's blood is not recommended because the levels of medication are usually low or nonexistent and negative effects are so rare. Your baby's blood may be tested only if there appears to be a serious problem related to medication, but this is extremely uncommon.

Help! My Pharmacist Warned Me against Taking Antidepressants While I Am Breastfeeding

Although many health care professionals have the best intentions when advising you against taking medication while nursing, they sometimes are not up to date on the data. Understandably, women get scared when a physician or health care professional tells them not to take a certain drug. They then go online to check the product information sheets or popular drug information resources, which say the same thing. This leaves them feeling confused, scared, and doubtful about who to believe.

The truth is that there are significant data about the safety of psychiatric medications during pregnancy and while breastfeeding, as described here. The data do not often make it into the information sheets you will get from your pharmacist about your pills or the CPS or PDR, mostly due to reasons of legal liability.

No drugs have been 100 percent approved by the US FDA or Health Canada for use in breastfeeding or during pregnancy, and many of the suggestions in this book are not officially sanctioned uses for these drugs by the drug manufacturer or national bodies that govern medications. However, their uses have been validated by medical research, and we know more about psychiatric drugs and their effects on pregnancy and lactation than we know about most other categories of drugs.

Treating Depression during Pregnancy

Unfortunately, pregnancy is not a glowing, happy time for all women. In fact, women who are pregnant have similar rates of depression compared to non-pregnant women. As you are aware, having depression or anxiety during pregnancy is a major risk factor for PPD and PPA. Let's talk about how you can manage depression if you get it while you are pregnant so that you can recover sufficiently to fully enjoy your pregnancy as well as the early days of having a new baby.

If you are depressed or anxious when you are pregnant, the self-care strategies discussed in Chapter 4 and talk therapy are excellent options for you to pursue. If your symptoms are not too bad and diminish when you make some changes and start therapy, that is great. However, if you continue to feel really depressed or very nervous, consider some additional treatment options, such as medication.

It is important that you treat your mood and anxiety during pregnancy not only to prevent PPD or PPA, but also because being severely depressed and pregnant can have serious negative consequences on your baby's health and well-being. Pregnant women who are depressed are more likely to abuse substances and are less likely to take good care of themselves while they are pregnant. Both of these factors can harm your baby. There is also evidence that severe depression increases the risk of having a miscarriage, high blood pressure, and of having a baby with health problems. There is so much that you can do to take charge of your depression while you are pregnant to prevent these problems.

If you decide to take an antidepressant while you are pregnant, it is important to understand the medication's effects on your baby in order to make informed decisions every step of the way.

There are four important factors to examine when considering medication during pregnancy. First, look at whether a medication increases the risk of a miscarriage or pregnancy loss. Second, look at the risk of organ malformation. Third, assess the effects on the newborn. Fourth, the long-term effects on the baby should be evaluated.

Some recent studies have shown that babies who were exposed to SSRIs *in utero* were more likely to be born one week early and to be admitted to special-care baby nurseries after birth. Other studies have shown conflicting results. There is controversial information about whether antidepressants are linked to an elevated rate of spontaneous abortion among women who take antidepressants of all types and much of the medical literature suggests that this happens because of a pregnant woman's depression or anxiety disorder rather than the medication.

Generally, TCAs, SSRIs, and SNRIs appear to be safe during pregnancy. After thousands of children were studied, there was no evidence of an increased risk of major organ malformations. In 2005, however, some disturbing information about paroxetine (Paxil) emerged. It seemed to be associated with heart defects and a rare condition called an omphalocele, which is a defect in the stomach wall that causes the intestines to protrude out of the body.

Although the numbers were very small, there was concern. The FDA moved paroxetine from a category C drug, which requires "caution when prescribing" and has "no positive evidence of risk in pregnancy," to a category D drug, which has "positive evidence of risk." A recently published study from The Motherisk Program in Toronto concluded that paroxetine is not associated with heart problems. Another study found that sertraline was associated with omphaloceles and a heart defect. And still another study created concern about all the SSRIs when it showed that when these medications are taken after 20 weeks of pregnancy, they can cause a rare but serious lung condition called persistent pulmonary hypertension of the newborn. Although some of the data remain concerning, the number of babies affected is minuscule and there are questions about the research methods that cast doubt on the direct link between the medications and this lung problem. It is important to note that other studies of thousands of babies who were exposed to SSRIs have not shown a significant increase in major malformations, including cardiac, brain, or lung defects. Also note that in the reports and studies that show negative effects of antidepressants, the number of babies negatively affected is still minuscule, despite being slightly elevated. Of course, you never want your baby to be the one who is negatively affected by a drug, but it is reassuring to see how small the absolute numbers are, and that safe data is continously emerging.

For a long time we have known that antidepressants can affect newborn babies. From 10-30 percent of newborns exposed to antidepressants later in pregnancy have "poor neonatal adaptation syndrome," which means that the baby experiences withdrawal symptoms or side effects, including breathing and feeding problems, and jitteriness. Although this can be alarming to new parents, these symptoms go away on their own within the first few days to the first week of the baby's life, and there have *never* been any long-term problems reported for these babies. If a newborn does appear to have symptoms, he or she should be observed for 48-72 hours prior to being discharged from the hospital.

In terms of long-term effects of antidepressant exposure *in utero*, there is limited but reassuring data. One study by Dr. Irene Nulman and colleagues at Sick Kids in Toronto that followed children up to seven years old who were exposed to fluoxetine *in utero* showed no differences in IQ, language, or behavioral development. Interestingly, this study found that if a mother continued to be depressed in the postpartum period and to have ongoing depressive episodes, the children had poorer IQ and language development. Another study, by Dr. Shaila Misri and colleagues in Vancouver found that children who were exposed to SSRIs did not have an increased risk of depression or anxiety or behavioral problems at age four. This study also showed that the mother's depression affected the children in a negative way.

So where does that leave us in terms of prescribing anti-depressants to pregnant women? The recent data raise some concerns. However, when the data are examined closely, there are conflicting results and problems with the methods of data collection, which makes it difficult to draw definite conclusions. It is important to remember that just because the use of anti-depressants is associated with problems does not mean that it causes these problems, and although SSRIs may be associated with some problems, it is essential to put this in perspective. The overall risks of taking an SSRI remain very low in terms of absolute numbers of babies affected.

The bottom line is that we do not know everything there is to know about the use of these drugs during pregnancy, and no one can guarantee zero risk. If you are experiencing severe depression, the problems associated with being depressed far outweigh the risks of using a scientifically studied drug under your doctor's supervision. The main concern is always for your health and your baby's health. Unfortunately, there is no perfect option when serious depression arises. However, there are solutions that will help you to get well and keep your baby very safe.

Should I Switch to a Safer Antidepressant While I Am Pregnant?

The answer to this question is a complicated one, and the principles of switching medication while breastfeeding are similar to the considerations you need to make during pregnancy. You need to discuss this with your physician and weigh the risks and benefits of the drug you are on with the risks of switching to a different drug. Again, if you have milder or easily treatable depression, it may be safer to change to a drug that has been well studied during pregnancy, such as fluoxetine. However, if you have a long history of more severe depression or anxiety and you cannot take some of the more well-studied drugs, staying on the drug that helps your illness may be the best choice for you. Again, there is no perfect answer and this is a complex balancing act that you and your doctor should discuss.

Should I Stop Taking Antidepressants in the Third Trimester?

In 2004, the US FDA and Health Canada issued warnings that using SSRIs and mirtazapine and venlafaxine during the third trimester of pregnancy could cause withdrawal symptoms or negative effects in newborn babies. Understandably, these announcements and the subsequent media buzz created much anxiety for pregnant women who were taking antidepressants. Many women abruptly stopped taking their medication without considering the consequences of doing this, and many more wondered if they should stop.

The reality is that these symptoms are the transient effects, as discussed in the last section, and are nothing new and nothing to be alarmed about. They are temporary symptoms and there is no evidence to suggest that they are a serious medical problem. No long-term cognitive, psychological, or behavioral consequences have ever been reported.

It is not a good idea for women who are being treated with an antidepressant during pregnancy to stop their medication in the third trimester or at any time toward the end of their pregnancy. Again, the treatment of depressed pregnant women requires a balancing act. The small potential of side effects for a newborn needs to be measured against the high risk of relapse for the woman during pregnancy and the postpartum period.

For women who have had a history of depression and require medication, there is a high relapse rate during pregnancy. According to one recent study by Dr. Lee Cohen and his colleagues at Harvard University in Boston, 43 percent of women with a history of serious depression developed depression while they were pregnant. Among those who stopped taking their medication during pregnancy, over 65 percent relapsed. Women who have had more than four episodes of depression and more than five years of illness with depression are the most likely to relapse during pregnancy. If you have a serious history of depression, it is not worth stopping your medication and taking on that risk.

Treatment for Women with Bipolar Disorder

If you have a history of bipolar disorder, it is ideal if you talk to your psychiatrist prior to getting pregnant in order to adjust your medications. If you are already pregnant and on a medication that is working well for you, changing your drug regimen can be risky because you may have a relapse either during pregnancy or in the postpartum period.

Women with a history of bipolar disorder who develop PPD are more complicated to treat because an antidepressant may not be right for them. When prescribed alone, an antidepressant may trigger a manic episode. Women with bipolar disorder often require treatment with a mood stabilizer, such as lithium, lamotrigine (Lamictal), valproic acid (Epival), or carbamazepine (Tegretol).

Until recently, lithium was regarded as dangerous during breastfeeding. Recently, there has been a variety of data showing that lithium enters the breast milk between 0 percent and 30 percent of the mother's dose. Under certain conditions, women who take lithium can breastfeed if their lithium level and the baby are closely monitored. If you breastfeed while taking lithium, do so under close physician supervision. You should also have access to a laboratory that can measure the baby's lithium level and do basic blood work, including kidney function tests and thyroid tests. Valproic acid and carbamazepine appear to be relatively safe for breastfeeding. Data show that these drugs enter breast milk at less than 5 percent of the mother's dose, so they are considered relatively safe for nursing mothers to take. Babies whose mothers take valproic acid should have their valproic acid drug levels tested, as well as their platelets and liver function. For carbamazepine, it is recommended that this drug level be tested in the baby's blood, as well as liver function and basic blood work. Regarding lamotrigine, there are many reports that show no problems when babies are exposed to this drug, but it can cause a dangerous rash as a side effect in adults, so babies need to be closely monitored for a rash and have their blood work done to test for liver function if they are breastfed. If you take any of these medications during pregnancy or while breastfeeding, please inform your pediatrician and request that your baby be closely monitored.

Finding the Truth Behind Scary News Stories

There is ongoing research about antidepressant safety during pregnancy and while breastfeeding. The results are frequently hot media topics. Negative results often trigger a flurry of concerned calls and raise anxiety levels.

Over the past few years, the Canadian and American governments' health agencies have issued warnings related to taking antidepressants during pregnancy. Although these warnings are meant to protect the public, they often generate significant fear and anxiety, and may have harmful effects because sometimes people make rash decisions on their own about their treatment plan.

In light of media reports and government communications, it is important that you have a strategy to deal with new information.

1. First, try not to panic. Call your physician and book an appointment to discuss your concerns.
2. With your doctor, discuss the recent information, weigh the pros and cons of your treatment, and see if you need to either change your medication or perhaps stop taking it.
3. Please do not stop taking your medication abruptly. This could lead to a return of your depression or anxiety as well as withdrawal symptoms.
4. Consult the following resources for excellent and up-to-date information about medication use during pregnancy and nursing:

- www.Motherisk.org
- http://toxnet.nlm.nih/gov (for breast feeding information go to LactMed section)
- www.reprotox.org (available by subscription)
- www.womensmentalhealth.com

Please also refer to the Resources section at the back of the book.

Other Treatments for PPD

Here are some other treatment options you mave have questions about:

Electroconvulsive Therapy (ECT)

ECT is a controversial treatment that often conjures up frightening images from *One Flew over the Cuckoo's Nest*. In reality, it is an excellent treatment for very severe depression, including depression with psychotic symptoms and very severe depression during pregnancy and in the postpartum period. ECT is used if someone is very ill and has not responded adequately to medications or cannot take medications or prefers not to, or if someone's physical health is jeopardized by depression (i.e., if someone is not eating or drinking).

ECT is thought to work because it delivers a seizure to the brain that affects chemicals in the brain and creates an antidepressant effect. ECT is usually done by a psychiatrist and an anesthetist together. A patient lies down and is then given an anesthetic to fall into a deep sleep, as well as a muscle relaxant. Electrodes are placed on the head, and brief electric shocks are sent into the brain, triggering a seizure. The body does not seize because of the muscle relaxant. The major side effects from ECT are confusion immediately after the treatment, which goes away, and sometimes memory loss that takes a few months to resolve.

ECT is a safe treatment that often helps someone feel better quickly and helps her stay well for a long time. It is by no means a first-choice treatment for someone with PPD, but can be extremely helpful in the rare situation when psychotherapy and medication do not work for extremely serious PPD or postpartum psychosis.

Hormones

Many women ask about taking estrogen and progesterone supplements to treat PPD or PPA. It makes sense to consider this idea since these illnesses often develop after hormone levels drop around delivery. Although some studies have looked at the use of estrogen to treat PPD, we do not know enough to recommend it at this time, and there may be serious side effects. Progesterone is not recommended because it might increase depression. More research needs to be done in this area before hormones can be considered a safe and effective treatment for PPD and PPA.

Natural Treatments and Dietary Supplements

It is understandable why some new mothers want to try natural treatments, such as herbal remedies for postpartum mental health concerns, particularly if they are breastfeeding. It is important to remember that even though natural remedies are available on the market, this does not mean that they are safe or effective. Unfortunately, we have even less information about natural treatments than we do about conventional medical therapies. Most herbal or natural treatments have not been examined as treatments for PPD specifically, and there is limited data about natural products and breastfeeding.

As a medical doctor and not a naturopath, my expertise is not in the prescription of naturopathic remedies and medicines. However, there is scientific evidence in support of some of these alternatives. But since these treatments have not been studied for PPD or PPA or for breastfeeding, they need to be approached with the same caution you would take for conventional medicines with limited data.

There are also some other things to think about before you take natural supplements. First, it can be difficult to know exactly the composition of the tablet you are taking. There can also be significant variability between brands and preparations. Most natural products are not regulated in the same way as prescription drugs. Also, these remedies must be taken with the same care and caution as any other drugs: They have real side effects and interactions. If you want to pursue these options, I suggest you contact a naturopathic doctor.

If you are already taking a natural remedy, please inform your doctor so that your treatment can be monitored and you can also discuss possible side effects and interactions with other medications.

The natural treatments described below are sometimes used to treat depression:

St. John's Wort (Hypericum)

Some medical studies have shown that St. John's wort is a useful treatment for mild or moderate depression. St. John's wort can have dangerous interactions with some prescription drugs and may compromise the efficacy and safety of other medications. Side effects include agitation, nausea, and skin sensitivity. St. John's wort has not been examined as a treatment for PPD and there is not enough data to suggest it is safe to take while breastfeeding.

S-adenosyl-L-methionine (SAM-e)

S-adenosyl-L-methionine or SAM-e (pronounced "Sammy") is an amino acid derivative. It has been hypothesized that SAM-e increases the availability of the neurotransmitters serotonin and dopamine. Studies have found that SAM-e is an effective treatment for depression in adults. It may have fewer side effects and works more quickly than conventional antidepressants. This is good news for adults suffering from depression, but SAM-e has not been studied as a treatment for PPD. Currently, there is no data about its passage into breast milk.

Omega-3 Fatty Acids

Omega-3 fatty acids are naturally occurring elements found primarily in fish. Pregnant and breastfeeding women may have low levels of these elements as they are naturally transferred to babies *in utero* and through breast milk. Omega-3 fatty acids have been looked at as a treatment for general depression and PPD. Current evidence cannot confirm that omega-3 fatty acids are an effective treatment of postpartum depression. However, there has been some research suggesting that when higher levels of omega-3 fatty acids are consumed by groups of women, rates of PPD are lower. Some data also suggests that omega-3 fatty acids may be useful to augment the effects of an antidepressant. Research in this area is ongoing.

It is currently safe and healthy, however, for you to eat regular portions of (lower-mercury-containing) fish such as sardines, herring, rainbow trout, salmon, canned light tuna, and canned mackerel to boost your omega-3 fatty acid levels, which can benefit your baby and your health.

After getting some answers and clarity about antidepressants and other medications, I hope that you will now feel reassured about taking medication if that's what you decide to do. The professional help and support you get from psychotherapy or medication will go a long way toward your recovery. The people you are close to can also be of tremendous value in helping you recover from PPD and PPA and stay well. In the next chapters, I will talk about how your partner, your family, and your friends can make a real difference for you and nurture your recovery.

Chapter 8

Weaving Your Web of Support

"She is a friend of mine.... The pieces I am, she gather them and give them back to me in all the right order."
—From Beloved *by Toni Morrison*

Now that you've begun your journey of recovery, you've made some significant changes to your sleep and routine, and you are dealing with your thoughts and emotions in a healthier way. You may have also established a relationship with a therapist and/or a physician and your treatment plan is coming together. In the meantime, the people in your life probably continue to ask you if and how they can help. Like most women, it may be very hard for you to answer that question; you may not know what to ask for or exactly what you need from others. More than anything, it may be really tough for you to ask for help at all. However, getting help from other people and having a robust support network is a significant part of recovering from PPD or PPA and a key to keeping you well. This means that when the current people in your life, and maybe even new contacts, rally around to help you in a meaningful way, this can make a big difference for your recovery from postpartum problems and your continued well-being.

Are you a member of the "I just can't ask other people for anything" club? I will talk about some of the barriers to getting the help you need and some effective ways to ask for help. Most new moms cite their partner as their closest connection and number one support. If you have PPD or PPA, your relationship with your partner may be under a great deal of strain. Study after study shows that your partner can be instrumental in helping you recover from PPD, and you obviously really want to get this relationship back on track. For this reason, I have written the next chapter specifically for the two of you. In the meantime, whether or not you are in a relationship (or if your partner is away for long stretches of time), the information in this chapter will help you create or boost your support system.

First, I will talk about how your difficulty asking for help is *not* helpful right now. Then I will talk about the types of support you need, and suggest some direct ways that you can get help from others.

You Really Do Need Support

For all new moms, having a sturdy support network will help make a smooth adjustment to parenting. If you have PPD or PPA, your support system can truly limit the impact from the bumps in the road and help you over the seemingly insurmountable challenges you face. In Chapter 2 you learned how having a bad or nonexistent support system can be a risk factor for PPD. In this chapter, you will learn how you can develop a healthy and helpful support group. We talk about a support "network" or "system" because one person alone cannot take care of all your needs. Different people can help you at different times and in different ways. A support network is essentially a group of people who may include your partner, family members, friends, coworkers, and even other new moms or other people you have just met, to whom you can turn for assistance and support at this time in your life. The support system that you create for yourself can consist of people who are both new and old in your life, as well as people you hire to help you out. Many studies have shown that people who have strong support networks and close relationships with others recover from depression more quickly, have fewer episodes of depression, and fewer physical illnesses. If you do not already have a strong and responsive support network, it is ideal if you can develop one to help you get through PPD or PPA. Since you may not know how to do that or what to ask for, I will make some suggestions about how you can do all these things in the pages to come.

Me, Ask for Help? No Way!

The real obstacle to building a successful support network often has little to do with a lack of available sources. It is more likely the result of a psychological block around the idea of asking for help, as well as the symptoms of PPD or PPA that keep you isolated. Let's take a look at why you may find it so difficult to ask for help even though you know you need it now more than ever.

It is interesting to note that this is the *third* time in this book that issues of shame and guilt may be preventing you from feeling well and enjoying motherhood. Once again, let's examine the deeply entrenched myths (which you may not even know that you believe in) that are hindering you from creating a solid support system. You may also find that this is an area worth exploring in therapy.

I Just Don't Want to Be around Anyone

Connecting to other people and reaching out is probably one of the last things you feel like doing right now. By now you know that isolation and withdrawal are symptoms of PPD and PPA. If you are like most moms with postpartum problems, the thought of talking to people is scary or irritating, and your illness makes you want to stay home alone and avoid the rest of the world. Depression and anxiety make you feel awkward in social situations and feel like others are judging you harshly. As you get better, these intense feelings of disliking other people and not wanting to be seen by anyone will subside. In the meantime, remember that while building a support network *may* entail socializing with new moms or other people, this is not the only thing it means. Developing your support network and getting help may at first mean asking others to assist you with specific chores or asking them to do errands for you and your baby. Please don't discount the idea of building a support network because you don't feel like being around people right now. Socializing can be an important part of your life and support network, but it does not have to happen until you are ready. In the meantime, there are many other ways that people can help you out.

I Don't Want Anyone to Know I Have PPD

You may worry that asking for help will alert others that something is "wrong" with you and you don't want anyone to know that you have PPD. Again, this is the stigma of mental illness and part of the myth of what new moms *should* be able to deal with. You have two options: First, you can ask for support and not disclose that you have PPD, because you have the right to keep this private. Second, you can tell someone about your experience with PPD, educate this person about your illness, and enlist his or her help. You may find that by telling those you are close to and whom you trust you will get even more warmth, reassurance, and help than you could have imagined. While you are teaching others all about your illness, you can also tell them that PPD is very treatable and you will recover.

I Should Be Able to Deal with Everything on My Own
Whether it is about acknowledging that you have PPD, getting
professional help for depression, taking medication, or turning
to others, you may feel that you have to be independent, self-
reliant, and self-sufficient. Or, if these *shoulds* are not coming
from within you, you may have other people reminding you
about how you *should* be managing on your own with your
new role and responsibilities.

Aubrey's mother could not understand why she continued
to ask her for help in taking care of the baby. She said, "When
I had you, I was all alone and I just took care of everything.
There is no reason why you should be any different." Kather-
ine's husband balked at her suggestion that she hire someone
to help her clean the house. He said, "You are at home all day,
this is your only job, and you should do it on your own." Our
culture values—or perhaps overvalues—independence and
self-sufficiency, which can be great qualities to have, but there
is a limit. Now is the time to ignore all the *shoulds* swirling
around inside of you and coming at you from others. Stop
shoulding on yourself! Having a new baby can be challenging,
and having PPD on top of that is definitely one of life's rougher
experiences. Now is the time to confront your notions of success and competency. Just watch yourself: See how the harsh,
self-critical feelings, such as inadequacy and guilt, arise when
you think about asking for help. Instead of letting these feelings
continue to keep you isolated and overwhelmed, consider how
relieved you would feel if you let others give you a hand or be
there for you in these difficult times.

I Haven't Done Anything to Deserve Help
This is a big issue for many women, particularly for those who
are depressed.

You may feel unworthy or undeserving of support. Once again, you have internalized one of the dominant myths about what good women *should* be able to do and what they deserve. Of course you deserve help. You would be there for your closest friends if they needed support. Don't fall prey to this myth, which will keep you isolated and alone.

I'm Usually the Helper, Not the One Who Is Helped

You may be uncomfortable receiving help because you are used to being the caregiver. Your *real* strength lies in recognizing that you need other people at this vulnerable time and letting them assist you. This may be foreign and uncomfortable for you. To make it a bit easier to ask for and actually accept help, remember that you will not be in this position forever. Also, other people often really want to be helpful. It makes them feel good about themselves, just as you feel satisfied and useful when helping someone in need.

Other People Won't Do Things the Way I Like Them Done

Yes, everyone does things differently. If you ask your partner to bathe your baby, it won't be done in the same way that you do it. Your best friend may not fold your laundry to your specifications, but think about what really matters most at this time. It matters that others can pitch in to ease your burden and care for you and your baby. Again, remind yourself that this is not forever, but that it really is good enough for *now*, and that is what counts.

I've Been Let Down by Others before When I Asked for Help

Many people have trouble asking for help because they think others will let them down. Since being let down is too painful, they avoid asking for help altogether to avoid the pain of disappointment. Of course it hurts when others don't come through and, unfortunately, this does happen. If you have this attitude about help-seeking, stop and think: first, notice your depressive extreme thinking: second, think about the people in your life who have been there for you in different ways and who have not let you down. Also, think outside the box about seeking new forms of support such as meeting new moms or hiring some helpers. Your support system does not have to be big to be effective; it just has to be good and reliable. Remember that just because you had a bad experience with asking for help in the past, does not mean that it will happen again.

If you experience any of the thinking patterns described above, notice when these thoughts come up. Note how you feel when you hold on to these ideas, and how they may keep you isolated and overwhelmed. Now is the time to realize that there is another way—that reaching out will ultimately feel good and will truly help you get through the postpartum period.

Figuring out What You Need

I have discussed some of the psychological obstacles between you and getting help, but you may be having a hard time figuring out what you really need and who to call on. Let's talk about the types of help that may be useful for you at this time.

There are different types of support that various people can offer you. Chapter 2 briefly discussed the varieties of support, but it is worth repeating this information here and going into a little more detail because understanding this is crucial to building a meaningful support system. Developing a new and strong support network is crucial for all new mothers, not only for those with PPD or PPA. If you have postpartum problems, it is even more important for you to turn to others.

Support comes in different forms and each type is important for meeting different needs. There is emotional support,
practical help, and information and advice. Examples of emotional support include your sister being there with a shoulder
to cry on, or a mom in your support group with whom you can
share PPD experiences so you will feel less alone. Someone
can offer you practical help by cleaning your house or preparing a meal for you and your family, or watch your baby while
you take a much-needed break. Your aunt, who is a nurse and
works the night shift, may be able to provide good baby-care
advice through the long nights, and your coworker, who just
had a baby, can offer tips about how to get your baby to stop
crying. You need each of these kinds of support, in some way
or another, to help you get through the postpartum period and
recover from PPD or PPA.

Emotional Support
You probably already know to whom you can turn for warmth
and love, and who you can trust with talking about PPD or PPA.
Hopefully your partner is one of your main supports in this area,
and I will talk more about this important relationship later. If
you can identify a few other key people to whom you can really
open up, please do that. If you find that connecting with other
people is a long-standing problem for you that is only made
worse with PPD, this is important to address in therapy.

When you are in the grip of serious PPD or PPA, you may
find that there are only one or two people you are comfortable
connecting with. That is fine for a short time, but as you heal,
you may find it helpful and enjoyable to expand your emotional
support system. You don't have to look only to the people you
already know to support you emotionally. Think about meeting
new women, either other new mothers or other women with
PPD. Serena was surprised how happy she felt after meeting

other mothers in her local park. She didn't share her experience of PPD with these new friends, but she felt that she was not alone in struggling to care for two little kids and the feelings of frustration she sometimes had with her partner. Just chatting and connecting with other women at the same stage of life broke her cycle of isolation and loneliness and helped her to feel much better.

Who should you tell?

Many women are pleasantly surprised by the reactions they get when they tell their friends and family that they have PPD or PPA. They realize how common postpartum problems really are when they start to talk about it. As Theresa said to me, "When you start to open up about what is really going on, you realize how many people you know that have gone through the same thing." You may find that telling your close friends and other people you trust is therapeutic. Your openness can lead to deeper connections with some friends and to new relationships with others. When Theresa told her friend Grace that she had PPD, Grace put her in touch with another friend, Lucy, who had PPD a year before. Lucy became an important source of support and advice for Theresa as she recovered.

Whether it is connecting with old friends and familiar relatives or meeting new people you feel comfortable with, the important thing is that you reach out and make a personal connection. Try to take care of your emotional needs on a daily basis.

Here are some other ideas for creating connections:

1. Call a close friend.
2. Invite someone you feel comfortable with to come over.
3. Create a play group with other new moms.
4. Go to a support group for moms with PPD.
5. Call your neighbors who have kids to make a play date.

6. Go online and join a community of other new moms or women with PPD.
7. If you have chosen to work with a doula or midwife through your pregnancy and childbirth, this person can often also provide great at-home emotional support in the postpartum period.

Practical Help

When it comes to thinking about practical support and help, many moms with PPD or PPA feel so overwhelmed that they are not sure what to ask for, or they just don't have the energy to write up a "to do" list for other people. To help you with this task, here is a list of practical things that you can ask other people to help you with:

Child-care needs
1. feed the baby
2. change the baby's diapers
3. bathe the baby
4. dress the baby
5. take the baby out so you can get some rest at home
6. stay with the baby so you can go out
7. stay with the baby so you can take a nap
8. arrange play dates or activities for your other children

Household needs
1. do the laundry
2. cook or order a meal
3. get groceries
4. clean the house
5. do some errands

Special needs
1. arrange for you to have a massage or spa treatment
2. rent a movie for you
3. drive you somewhere you need or want to be
4. pick up something for you
5. answer your phone or doorbell while you are sleeping
6. let you sleep—take over night feeding so you can sleep longer

If you don't have people in your life who can meet some of these needs, you may want to consider hiring a helping hand, such as someone to help with cooking, cleaning, laundry, or child care during the first few weeks or months.

Information and Advice

In terms of informational support or advice, you are likely to know where to turn to and who you can talk to. Some useful supports in this area may include a friend who has recently had a baby, your pediatrician, your therapist, your doctor, your doula or lactation consultant if you have them, members of your religious or cultural group, or neighbors. If you are looking for additional information, please check the Resources section at the back of this book for more ideas.

Now make your own list of the types of help you need and who you can contact for help:

Type of Support	Name of Person #1	Name of Person #2	Name of Person #3
Emotional needs			
Practical help			
Information/advice			

Seeking Support from Your Own Home: Using the Phone or Internet

Many new moms find that it is hard to get out of the house with a young baby. Either the weather is too cold, or too hot, or the baby is sleeping, or they are too tired or just cannot be bothered with getting themselves, their baby, and the diaper bag organized. For women with depression or anxiety, the tendency to withdraw from the world and to be fearful of going out increases their isolation. For this reason, many women find that the phone and the Internet are essential lifelines.

Calling friends or family members is a good place to start connecting if you are depressed and reluctant to see other people. There are also postpartum hotlines that you can call for information and support.

On the Internet, you can find support groups for women who have PPD or PPA. There are social networking sites that bring together women with depression and anxiety. On these Web sites, women share stories and treatment information. There are chat rooms and other discussion groups or Listservs that you can join. These online services allow you to connect with other women who also have postpartum illnesses. You may find it helpful to read about other women's experiences with motherhood or with PPD or PPA. There are many blogs written by moms who have or have had PPD or PPA, as well as Web sites that can offer information.

As with all support and information that you find, you need to assess the validity of online sources. Please avoid changing your treatment plan on your own or because of the advice of someone you meet online. It is always best to discuss your plans with your health care provider. However, the Internet can still be a powerful vehicle for you to connect with other women and find support and information that you may not find elsewhere or easily access. Please turn to the Resources section at the back of this book to find more information about telephone hotlines and reliable online sources.

What about my other children?

Your relationship with your older kids is very important to you. If you have PPD or PPA, you probably find it hard to be the kind of mom you want to be for your other children. While you are recovering:

1. **Keep your children's lives as normal as possible**
   Although it may be hard for you to continue parenting your older children as you usually do, try to keep their lives as routine as possible. Enlist the help of your partner and your support system to keep your other kids active outside of the home and caught up with school or activities. The more they can be involved with things that make them feel good and the more they can maintain their routine, the less your depression will impact them. Your kids might sense that you are depressed and that all is not perfect, but if their lives are the same as usual, they can be happily distracted as you work toward wellness.

2. **Use teamwork**
   Work together as a team to meet your kids' needs: Ask your partner to compensate for your limitations right now. In general, this is an important parenting principle, but it is even more essential when you are not at your best. In Chapter 9 I will discuss your relationship with your partner in detail.

3. **Talk to your kids**
   Kids pick up on their parents' moods and can sense when their mom is not quite herself. They may get worried if they see you crying a lot and may wonder why you aren't spending as much time with them. Letting kids know (especially older kids who can understand) that you are sick and not feeling well is a great idea. You can say something as simple and straightforward as: "You're right, I have been upset and tired lately. I have not been feeling well." If their observations are validated, children are less likely to feel scared or fear that your unhappiness is their fault. Also, don't forget to emphasize to the kids that you are getting help and will feel better soon. This way they will know that the adults in the family are taking charge and that you will be all right. And, of course, reinforcing how much you love them, despite not feeling well, goes a long way.

How to Ask for What You Need

Now that we have cleared away some of the barriers to asking for help and you have thought about building a winning support system, let's talk about how to ask for help in a way that will ensure that you get what you need.

These tips will help you to communicate your needs and will make the process of asking for help go more smoothly. You can use these ideas for talking to your partner or to anyone else you turn to.

1. *Let others know exactly what you want*

   Although clarity may not be your number one asset these days, be very explicit and direct about what you need and want done. The more specific and clear you are with your wishes, needs, and instructions, the more likely others will be able to help you in a way that is meaningful to you. Start with one specific task and define the task.

2. *Try to be calm*

   When you are depressed, sleep deprived, and overwhelmed, politeness is not at the forefront of your mind. In fact, you probably have a much shorter wick than usual. Though the last thing in the world you may want to do is worry about self-restraint, staying calm is helpful in getting communication rolling and keeping it on the right track.

3. *Try not to criticize*

   Giving up the reins of control can be hard, whether it is asking someone to care for your baby or clean your house. If someone does not do something in quite the way you would like it done, take a deep breath, step back, and try to let go. Although it may certainly be challenging, don't take out your frustration and irritation on whoever is helping. Try to value the fact that you are not the one who needs to get these tasks done.

4. *Show thanks and appreciation*

When you are feeling depressed, it can be hard to thank the people who are helping you. However, this is worth remembering and worth the effort. Although you need not be effusive with your thanks, and although you are not in a position to give much back right now, people feel really good when they are thanked and appreciated. They are also more likely to want to continue to help.

In this chapter I discussed the obstacles that stand in the way of building your support network. I talked about who can assist you with your diverse needs, and how to get the help you want. I discussed building a secure web that will comfort and sustain you through the difficult days of PPD or PPA. No matter what circumstances you find yourself in or where you live, there are resources that are available to you. It is well worth making the effort to organize and orchestrate your vital support network. In the next chapter, I will explore the relationship that is likely at the epicenter of your web: your relationship with your partner.

Chapter 9

Just the Two of You:
The Postpartum Partnership

This chapter is for you and your partner. The two of you should read it. It is addressed to both of you, as if I were speaking to you in my office for a session together.

At the end of the day, when you shut your front door, you and your partner remain at the center of your life and at the core of your growing family. How will you become a team to get through the experience of having a baby and recovering from PPD or PPA together? You may turn to your partner and wonder what happened to your once-stable and enjoyable relationship, which has deteriorated since your baby was born. The first exciting year of your baby's life may be the hardest and most painful one for your relationship. Almost every couple argues more after the arrival of a baby. Money, parenting tactics, and who contributes more to the family are all common things for new parents to argue about. Both you and your partner feel tired and anxious about your new role, and you each go into personal survival mode. When you are not taking care of the baby or trying to figure out how to parent, you are each trying to take care of yourself. You are probably feeling quite alone. Many couples face these issues after having a baby. Under the added burden of PPD or PPA, your relationship with your partner will be even further challenged. In this situation, inertia often takes over and nurturing your relationship takes a backseat to the huge demands of caring for your new baby and dealing with postpartum problems. Read on to learn how the two of you can break through the isolation and develop an even stronger bond.

You already know that having a difficult relationship with your partner is a risk factor for PPD. Relationship strain can also make depression worse and longer lasting. I don't have to tell you how incredibly difficult it is for both partners when you are new parents, especially when a new mom is dealing with PPD. Not only do even the most basic of assumptions and hopes that you had about being new parents go entirely out the window, but both of you lose one of the few remaining steadfast sources of joy and stability: each other.

At the same time, developing a solid team with your partner will help limit the impact of PPD and PPA and can definitely accelerate recovery. Building a treatment plan as a team, and figuring out how you can each play a part in the solution is important. There is a lot of evidence to show that your partner can have a powerful and positive influence over your healing.

Teamwork can bring you even closer together as you work to recover from PPD or PPA. As each of you learns to talk more clearly and to provide empathy and mutual support, you will do really well as a couple and come through this time with a new level of intimacy. Your children will also reap the benefits of your improved partnership.

In this chapter, I will help you understand some of the issues that may be stressing one of the most valuable assets to recovery from PPD or PPA—your relationship with your partner. I will also discuss how you can come together as a strong unit and get through your illness.

When I see couples with postpartum problems, they often wonder what to say or not say to one another, and how to enlist each other's help and support. To address these questions and concerns, I have written letters to each of you from the other person. These letters state clearly what each of you is likely feeling and experiencing. This will help the other person understand where you are coming from. The letters also describe how your partner would like you to respond to him or her. I hope the letters help to reduce some of the confusion and perhaps resentment that may be coming between you as you each struggle to understand the other's behavior. Often when members of a couple can let each other know how they feel, it can go a long way toward improving their relationship and bring them closer. At the end of the chapter, I will suggest some ways that you two can begin to talk about things in a more productive way to strengthen your relationship as it weathers the wild postpartum storm. With this insight and these new ideas, the two of you can begin to support one another in a meaningful and helpful way.

A Letter to Your Partner

Dear Partner,

I am going through this horrible experience and I need you to be by my side. There are some things I would like to share with you to help you understand how I'm feeling. I know I seem negative toward you and dismiss your efforts sometimes. There are some things I need to ask of you, so that we can carry on and continue to grow as a family.

I Want You to Understand How I Feel and to Learn about PPD/PPA

I think I have assumed, incorrectly, that you know what it is like to struggle with PPD or PPA, but now I realize that you can't possibly know. You have never had this illness and you can't read my mind. I need to start talking with you openly about how I feel. What I want more than anything is for you to listen to what I am going through and to help me make some sense of this. Please start by reading Chapter 3 of this book, which covers the signs and symptoms of depression and anxiety. This will help you see that my behavior and some of my thoughts are part of a real illness. It would be so helpful to me if you could understand the ins and outs of this illness. It is a very treatable problem and I am working hard to get better to care for our little baby, but recovery will take some time. I hope you understand that I am truly unwell right now and that I want to be both a great mom and a caring partner for you.

I want to teach you about PPD or PPA and to point you toward other good sources of information, because learning about it and how it is treated will help you to stay positive and informed (and not become pessimistic when things feel like they are progressing slowly). You have the potential to be the greatest support and the most important motivator in my life right now, so please take on this task.

Be Part of My Treatment Plan and Support My Treatment Decisions

Let's create a treatment plan together and both stay involved in it. It is never too late for you to get involved. Please come with me to some of my appointments to meet the people who are helping me, to learn about the treatments I am getting, and to take the opportunity to raise your questions or concerns. If you want to, you can probably even book some private time with the professionals I am seeing and ask them any questions that you have about me or my treatment, or about how you can cope with what our family is going through.

Be Patient with My Illness and Recovery Progress

I know that you have never seen me like this and thank goodness for that. If you aren't depressed and have never been depressed, it can be entirely foreign and hard to understand. You keep telling me to "just be happy" because I have so much to be thankful for, which is so true. But that comment is actually hurtful and I feel guilty when I hear you say things like that. If I could "just snap out of this," believe me, I would!

The treatment of PPD or PPA takes time. I wish that I could be better after my first therapy session or after taking one week of medication. However, the reality is that improvement may be slow and uneven and there may be bad days. We both wish I would feel better immediately, but we need to be realistic and to know that even though I am working hard to get better, it won't happen overnight. But I will get better.

Please stay hopeful and optimistic for me and with me. And let me know if you see progress. When you are paying attention and looking out for me, I feel so comforted.

As Hard as This May Be for You, I Need You to Accept This

I know I just asked you to be optimistic, but at the same time, please don't *push* me to be better and back to normal immediately. It may seem as if I am asking you to walk a tightrope, but there is a sweet spot between being supportive and accepting that this is where I am right now. If you can accept that I have PPD or PPA and that I am doing what I can to be healthy, I think it would help speed up my recovery.

I know you have been trying to rationalize this problem, but rationalization won't help me out of depression and anxiety. Explaining to me why I *shouldn't* feel the way I feel or why it makes no sense for me to be down worried is not helpful. If I could feel better immediately, I would. Through this process, I have learned that depression and anxiety take over and color how I think. I guess I am really asking you to tell me that you know I feel badly and that you can see I am suffering.

Telling Me What to Do Doesn't Work

Telling me how I should spend my days or what else I need to do to get better isn't helpful. You know that neither of us likes to be told what to do. And please don't remind me what you would do if you were in my situation.

Again, I know you are trying to say and do the right thing. At this point, I need you to support me in doing things that will help me feel good. Sometimes I dismiss your ideas because I have to create my own.

The Little Things Mean So Much

One of the main reasons I love to be with you is because you can be so supportive of me. Please continue to be so. I would love to hear your praise. If I seem more confident in taking care of our baby, tell me. If I make you a meal that is tasty, let me know how much you appreciate it. As you know, depression and anxiety have sapped my confidence, so external validation goes a long way for me now. And please keep telling me that you love me and that you will stick by my side. A cup of tea in bed, a surprise treat, or an acknowledgment all remind me that you are thinking of me.

This Is Not Your Fault and You Can't Just Fix This

Many partners want to fix each other when something goes wrong, and we are no different. Once you know a bit about PPD or PPA and the recovery process, you will know that this is caused by a combination of biological, psychological, and social factors, and it is not your fault or mine. There is no magic-bullet solution, but recovery will come from all the steps I have taken on my own and the ones we are taking as a team. Try not to get frustrated with me or the process. Let's be patient and take these small steps forward together.

A "To Do" List

There are so many concrete ways in which I would really appreciate your support and help. I'm trying to be clear about what I need. I know it is not fair for me to get frustrated that you can't read my mind or instinctively "just know" what to do. Please see the list in Chapter 8 for some suggestions, and also let's get more outside help, either from the people in our life or from someone we hire to help us take care of ourselves, our home, and our family.

As a partner, when do you take charge?

1. If your partner is not caring for herself or the baby
2. If your partner seems to be acting strangely or saying unusual things
3. If your partner is talking about hurting herself, the baby, or anyone else

In these situations, your partner may not want to get help, and she may resist it. However, if she is severely ill, she may be incapable of making good decisions and you need to take charge and manage the situation. Please see page 78 to learn how to deal with these emergencies.

A Letter From Your Partner

Dear Partner,

Seeing you suffering with PPD or PPA has been terrible. I feel so helpless, worried, and frightened for you. I also feel so alone. I want you to be better soon so that I can have my partner back. I miss you. I hope we can get on soon with parenting our baby together and being the happy family we dreamed about. My letter to you is not meant to make you feel badly or feel guilty, but I want you to know where I am coming from and what I am also going through. How can we be a team to deal with PPD or PPA together? Here are a few things I want you to understand about my experience.

I'm Also Working through This Big Life Change

I never could have imagined how life-altering having a baby and becoming a parent really is. I'm mystified about how to be a parent and it's taking me time to adjust. I sometimes have no idea what to do with our baby and it is terrifying. I guess I thought I would learn a lot from you as you took the driver's seat for the first little while, and now I am shocked and a bit overwhelmed to find that I am the one in charge. My friends told me that I would be three months behind you when it comes to accepting pregnancy and being prepared for a baby, and it seemed funny at the time. But now that you have PPD /PPA, it isn't funny at all. I feel scared and overwhelmed trying to take care of the baby and you at the same time.

Please Understand That I'm Caught between Work and Home

I feel pulled in so many different directions right now. I know I need to be around more to take care of you and our baby, but I am really stressed out about my job. I never planned to take this much time off work or to be called away from work so often. Now that we are more dependent on my income alone, I feel stressed out when I have to miss work and I worry about doing a good job. We need for me to keep my job and continue to support our family. I feel as if I am needed or expected to be in two places at once, but I am not able to do anything well or make anyone happy.

I Don't Know How to Handle This Situation

I think I'm supposed to be able to handle everything, but I'm pretty short on ideas as to what to do now. I've never experienced anything like this in my life. I was sensing for a while that things were not quite right for you, but I didn't know how to talk to you about it. When I tried to broach this, I guess I didn't express myself very well and you felt I was criticizing you. I'm not quite sure what I can do to be helpful to you now. I seem to always say the wrong things or not do the right things. It feels as if I'm walking on eggshells in our own home. It's hard when you are critical and angry with me. I thought I was doing the best I could to be helpful. I wish you could tell me clearly what you need from me and how I can help you get better, and if you are not sure, perhaps we can ask a professional to guide us.

> **How to care for yourself when your partner has PPD:**
>
> 1. First, start by realizing that you *need* to care for yourself too.
> 2. Realize that it is okay to have negative feelings and to feel upset and disappointed that your partner has PPD or PPA.
> 3. Get help for yourself, and find someone to talk to.
> 4. Join a support group for new parents (see Resources section).
> 5. Ask your family or friends to help out so you can also have a break.

Depression and the other parent:

- If your partner has PPD, you are also at higher risk of depression.
- Your depression may start later in the year after your baby is born.
- The signs and symptoms can be the same, but men are more likely to feel intense anger, act aggressively, and have substance-abuse problems when they are depressed or anxious.
- Take steps to get professional help, as described in Chapter 5.

A Team Approach: How You and Your Partner Can Get through This

Every good relationship requires attention and hard work to sustain it, and this is particularly true for those under the strain of PPD or PPA. When the dark clouds begin to lift, it is essential to nurture and revitalize your connection to one another. Here are some things that you and your partner can do to improve your relationship:

1. Find Time to Be Alone as a Couple

Spending time together is essential for nurturing your relationship. This might sound like advice that is too simple for you to take seriously. Ilana felt the same way. She initially dismissed this suggestion, but a few weeks later, Ilana confessed: "I took your advice and asked Seth to go out for dinner, alone, without the kids. I planned a night out. Nothing fancy, we just went around the corner to a local burger place. It was only a little thing, but it felt like a big thing. It was so easy, but it made such a big difference for Seth and me, and he kept thanking me too."

After Liz had her first date night with Paul, she told me: "Wow, I now remember why I really love Paul and why I married him in the first place. With everything going on in our lives, I had forgotten all that."

You may not feel prepared to leave your baby with another caregiver right away or to be apart from your baby, but you can still carve out time at home together. Make sure you and your partner are focused on one another and are not checking e-mail, your BlackBerries, or answering the phone. Sit down together and pay attention to each other.

As your baby gets a bit older, you may venture out of the house or out on dates for an evening or overnight. One couple, Patty and Rob, asked their parents to babysit for one night each month so they could go to a local hotel room and enjoy a baby-free soiree. Time together, just the two of you, may not spontaneously happen during these first few years of parenthood, so schedule it and then protect it.

2. Limit How Much You Talk about PPD or PPA
Obviously, going through depression and anxiety is very consuming and you are really struggling to get better. Finding even small segments of time to talk about other things together can be really important and enjoyable.

3. Let's Talk about Sex
Most new parents find that their sex lives change drastically when they have a new baby. Many couples don't make love for the first seven or eight weeks after the baby is born, and they have sex 40 percent less frequently in the following year. With PPD or PPA, your sexual relationship is likely to become even more complicated. You may be still recovering from delivery, your hormones may be causing vaginal dryness, or you might

feel self-conscious about your postpartum body, distracted by your baby or worried about being interrupted by noisy children. As discussed previously, depression or anxiety can reduce your libido, and if you are taking an antidepressant, unpleasant sexual side effects can be part of the package. With these factors stacked against you, lovemaking may not be something you are too keen on right now. Hopefully, you can explain all this to your partner and have his or her support. It may take some time until you are able to rekindle your sexual relationship. In the meantime, be sure to talk openly (and maybe even share some laughs) about your sex life, as awkward as it may feel. Reassure your partner that this is not a personal rejection of him or her. Suggest ways you can physically connect, such as hugging, massage, or cuddling, that feel more comfortable right now. Spending quiet, intimate time together, even if you are not making love, can go a long way toward helping you and your partner stay close. As your PPD or PPA improves and your body recovers from delivery, your sex life can get back on track.

4. Get Outside Help If You Need It

If you are having fights every time you try to talk or if it feels that you and your partner are growing further apart and you don't know how to find your way back to a common ground, get some help. A marital therapist can help you learn to communicate more effectively, and you might find it useful to have a neutral third party to guide your conversations. More detailed information about couples therapy was described in Chapter 6. Couples are often fearful or embarrassed about seeing a therapist. Many couples view couples therapy as the first step toward the end of the relationship. In fact, therapy is a powerful step toward connection and maturity in a relationship.

What Can I Say? : Communicating With Your Partner

Here are some ideas to help you and your partner *really* talk to one another. Before you try these, think about the relationship challenges and issues that the two of you have already encountered and overcome as a couple. You have already been successful in dealing with problems together. As you are experiencing this difficulty, you may not realize that you can use what has worked previously for your partnership. At the same time, you might find that some of the ways you normally communicate are not working so well under the intense stress you are now both experiencing. Here are some communication suggestions to try as you are finding your way together. Experiment with these ideas and see what works for you. Even if you can make one little change, you will feel happier, better understood, and more attuned to your other half.

1. The Right Time and the Right Place

Set yourselves up for success by making a date to talk. Limit distractions and interruptions so that you and your partner can focus on each other and on the conversation. By having an established time and date, you limit the likelihood that emotions will run high, so you can address the issues at hand rationally and clearly, rather than with anger and frustration. Planning ahead can help to ensure that you are both in the right frame of mind to have a serious talk. When you are rushing to get to work or bathing the baby while your toddler is tugging at your pant leg, it is not an ideal time. At these awkward and overwhelming times, it is much less likely that you will be able to have a productive and respectful conversation. In these moments, agree to a time that will be better for both of you and then put the issue aside until then.

2. Be Clear: Define a Problem

Once the two of you have come together at a good time to talk, start by being as specific as possible when deciding what you want to discuss. Pick one issue at a time and address only that issue. When too many issues are on the table, it is a surefire recipe for hurt feelings and for feeling unresolved after the conversation.

If you are bothered by the fact that you have to get up to feed your baby while your partner sleeps in every morning, focus on just that. Instead of saying: "You never do anything around here." You can try a more effective approach: "I need your help in the mornings with Ava, so let's discuss this."

3. Avoid Blame and Criticism

Blaming or criticizing are not the best ways to approach a conversation, but they can be incredibly hard to avoid, especially when you are under so much stress and are not feeling good about yourself. Even if you are working toward owning the problem, it is easy to start blaming: "You know I'm depressed, so why are you not doing anything to help me?" Blaming could well lead to escalating anger and lashing out, leaving you both feeling more helpless and less understood.

Instead, try talking about how you feel about something and how it is affecting you. So, continuing on the example started above, you can say: "I feel upset when I wake up every morning to feed Ava because all these early mornings are taking a toll on me and I am finding it hard to function."

While you may be tempted to believe that your partner is responsible for your misery or your problems at the time, if you can talk about how *you* feel and how your partner's behavior affects you, you're more likely to communicate effectively and get the empathy that you need. Notice the difference in the outcome when you use blaming versus talking about how you feel. Notice how the conversations feel different and how you and your partner react to each approach. Hopefully, instead of pointing fingers at each other, you will be holding hands.

4. Stay Focused on the Now

Did you ever notice how tempting it is to throw every griev-ance, past and present, into the mix, once the door is open? "You know I'm exhausted, so why can't you just get up and help me? Why do I *always* have to do everything around here?" For a few seconds, it feels cathartic and you feel powerful, but then your partner will likely get angry, disagree with you, and go on the offensive. More and more issues get thrown on the table, and hurt feelings and name-calling fall into the mix. The issues become larger than life and feel insurmountable. Instead, try to limit yourself to the topic *du jour*. This will lead to a more productive and respectful conversation. Although it can be hard to stay focused on one present issue, part of you already knows that if you blame, dredge up the past, and demand universal behavioral changes, not much will be resolved. For a better outcome, try to describe the behavior that irritates you by using the facts in the here and now: "I am upset that every morning I have to get up to feed Ava and I would like you to help me out." This statement helps you stay in the present mo-ment, and targets the issue at hand.

5. Get to Know Your Full Range of Feelings

When you are depressed, anxious, easily irritated, and upset, it can be hard not to let the anger color everything you are trying to express or request. For example, Melissa was really upset that Colin was planning to go to a bachelor party on Saturday night, leaving her alone at home with the baby. She said, "How can you think about leaving me when I'm having such a hard time? You're so selfish and you care only about your buddies. You don't care about me or the baby." This type of statement, called "dumping," happens when you yell, blame, and accuse out of anger. You may notice how unlikely you are to get the support you need with this approach. Anger is usually a cover for hurt feelings. It can be hard to be aware of and to express the feelings beneath the anger, but they are precisely what need to come out and where quality communication begins.

Instead, Melissa can introduce all of her feelings into the conversation by saying: "I'm *scared* that I am going to be alone with the baby for 24 full hours because I'm *worried* that I won't know how to care for him and that I will feel so *lonely*. And part of me is *envious* of you going away with your friends and having so much fun with them. I *fear* that you won't want to come home after such a great night away because it has been so rough here since the baby was born." You can see that this really reveals all of Melissa's emotions in the moment and Colin has the opportunity to hear how she is feeling beneath her anger. He is much more likely to be compassionate and to engage in a meaningful conversation this way.

6. Can You Read My Mind?

Another huge pitfall for many couples is assuming that the other person can and should read their mind. Other people fall into the trap of assuming that if they have told their partner something once, the other person will remember, and then if they forget, that means they don't really care. When you are talking to your partner, pay attention to your assumptions. Also pay attention to the expectations you have of him or her. Do you expect your partner to know something without you having to say it? Do you conclude that your partner doesn't love you if he or she has forgotten to do something? To get the most out of communication with your partner, be explicit about what you think, feel, and need. Don't assume that your partner knows you are upset about something until you actually say so. Also watch out for the "all or nothing" thinking or any other negative thinking patterns that were described in Chapter 4. You might want to review these and see if they are cropping up in your interactions with your significant other.

7. Be Direct: Express What You Need

If you have an idea about how you want something to happen or about the type of solution you want, say so. When you offer a solution, be clear and specific about behavioral changes that you would like to see. Set your partner up for success by asking for specific changes that he or she will know how to do. An ineffective approach would be to say: "You need to be more thoughtful and considerate and to contribute more to the running of this household and to the care of our baby." What's wrong with this statement? It uses anger and admonishing statements, is vague, and makes far too many sweeping demands. However, an effective way to approach this might be to say: "Let's each get up on alternating mornings to take care of Ava. That way there will be no surprises and the burden is shared equally between us. Will you help me try this?"

Often the issue you are discussing won't have a clear and straightforward solution. If you can't agree on an answer right away, it is okay to disagree for the time being and set up another time to continue the discussion. Sometimes you don't need a concrete solution, but you might be surprised that you feel better just by being heard and understood.

8. Learn How to Listen

It's not only what you say and how you say things that will improve your communication. It's also about listening to one another with respect and acceptance. Really listening to what your partner is going through, even if it doesn't make sense to you or seems totally irrational, is one of the most important things you can do right now. Listening without judgment is one of the toughest skills to learn. When you are really listening, you are open to your partner's emotions and experience. You do not need to correct or argue or try to defend yourself or even try to change him or her. Watch yourself to see if you can do this. Give it a go and notice how your partner reacts to you when you genuinely listen to him or her.

9. Take Your Time or Take a Time-out

Sometimes a conversation gets derailed when things are said too quickly in the heat of an argument. Emotions take over and you may regret some of the hurtful things you say. If your conversation has exploded and you are getting nowhere, you may wish to give yourselves a time-out. Yes, a time-out is a good technique for adults too! You may not need to send yourself to your room to cool off, but take a break from the intensity of the conversation. Agree to return to talking after a certain period of time, maybe 10 or 20 minutes. Take a breather, regroup, and return to try again.

These are particularly good strategies to build your team. They will help you on the rough seas of early parenthood under the cloud of PPD.

"What's Gonna Work? Teamwork!"

The kids in the park who sing this little ditty are offering great advice. Once you have heard where your partner is coming from, reflected on how he or she is feeling, and what your partner needs from you, you can actively try to do things differently and be there for each other in a new way. At the same time, this will help the postpartum problems fade into the background. This teamwork is such an important part of your treatment plan. You and your partner have chosen to be together for many good reasons. Successfully confronting PPD or PPA as a team will make you much better parents, strengthen your bond, and deepen your connection to one another. The two of you will be in an enviable position to manage almost any curveball that life throws your way. In the next chapter, I will discuss how you can build your family life and your future together as the shadow of PPD or PPA recedes.

Chapter 10

Moving On

If you are going through hell, keep going.
—Winston Churchill

You have really come a very long way. Now that you have your own treatment plan and supports in place and you are feeling more like yourself again, you are in recovery mode. Congratulations on coming this far—you have kept on going through the hell of PPD or PPA, and now you can see the light.

The Other Side: Recovering from PPD or PPA

If you've had a minor bout of depression or anxiety, recovery should occur rather quickly and smoothly. Recovering from a lengthy and more serious episode of depression or anxiety may take a while longer, but it will happen. It's impossible to say exactly how much time it will take for you to recover fully because everyone is different, and people improve at different rates. Rest assured that you will get well again and be stronger than ever. I have never met anyone who has not recovered from postpartum problems.

When you are feeling so much better, you might take

inventory of your life and think about your future from the excited perspective of a happier and healthier new mom. I have discussed how you and your partner can become a stronger unit, and you are probably wondering how you can continue to build your relationship with your baby. In this chapter, I will talk about how to do this proactively. I will also give you a heads-up about what you might experience along the road to recovery, and how to stay healthy once you are there.

Baby Love: Connecting With Your Baby

One of the biggest reasons that you have taken the courageous and strong steps to get well is for your sweet baby. You want to be the very best mom that you can be, and addressing your PPD or PPA is exactly the right place to start. The steps you have already taken toward recovery will enable you to build a close and loving relationship with your little one and prepare your baby for a happy, healthy life.

Here are some ways to strengthen your connection with your baby:

1. Smile and the World Smiles back at You

Once your depression and anxiety diminish, it will be much easier to pay attention to your baby and to smile from your heart, especially when you see that wide, gummy grin. Babies learn that the world is a safe place when those who care for them are responsive to their emotions and needs. Before they learn to speak, babies communicate through sounds, cries, facial expressions, and physical movements. When parents pay close attention to a baby's cues, the baby can begin to trust and feel comforted. If your baby is smiling, smile back. If your baby is crying, try to soothe him or her. If your baby is looking away and wants quiet time, let your child be. Of course, you will not always be able to meet your child's needs exactly, but if you can do so much of the time, you are doing a great job.

2. Goo-goo: Talking to Your Baby

Even when your baby is still very young, she or he is ready and eager to interact with you. Now that you are feeling well, you too will feel eager. Look at your baby, open your mouth, and stick out your tongue. Watch your baby's reaction. Your baby is listening to you from the start, so let the babbling begin.

You can chat with your baby about what she or he is doing and about what you are doing. For example, you can say: "Mommy is waving to baby." Or "Mommy is sitting with baby." Or "Baby is smiling at Mommy." You can even turn your commentary into a song. Yes, it may sound strange at first, but it gets easier with practise. The conversation does not have to make a lot of sense to you or to anyone who happens to be eavesdropping, but it makes a huge impact on your baby. Margaret was really anxious to start talking to her baby. She felt awkward and didn't know what to say at first. Her solution? She sat down on the floor beside her son, puffed out her cheeks, and said, "Poof!" Both she and the baby started to giggle. She was surprised how great she felt after this and how happy her baby seemed too.

Reading to your baby is another great thing to do. Your child may try to chew the book and probably can't sit through a full story, but he or she is listening to your voice and loving being with you.

3. Just You and Me, Baby

Lying on the floor, patting your baby, and smiling at one another is a great way to spend time with your newborn. Teach your baby how to play with toys. Roll in the grass with your little one. Just spending time together is a great way to connect and strengthen your bond.

What to Expect on the Road to Recovery

I've been fortunate enough to have been a part of the recovery process for hundreds and hundreds of women. Every woman gets well at her own pace, but the wonderful thing is that everyone does get well! Before we go our separate ways, let's take a look at some of the most common paths of recovering from PPD or PPA. These are worries, pressures, and anxieties that occur, and also some life changes that may have an impact on you. The more you know about what to expect (and the more you share with your partner and other major supports), the better equipped you will be to get back to normal quickly.

1. On the Road Again

Recovery from depression is not perfectly smooth, unfortunately. You might feel good for a few days, then great for a week, and then you may have a few difficult days.

It can be hard for women recovering from PPD to know whether a bad day is just a bad day or if it means that depression is returning. And trying to distinguish between the two can create anxiety. If you have a day or two or three that are rough, after feeling well for a while, you may be terrified that a long spiral downward has begun again. This fear is especially common, and especially frightening, in the early days of recovery. In this case, notice how your extreme thinking may be taking over. Remember, just because one day is bad it does not mean that tomorrow will be hard or that you are "slipping." It might just be a bad day. Bad days are a normal part of life and of the recovery process.

> A few tough hours or days do not mean you are depressed again.

You have already developed excellent ways to get your mind-set and feelings back on track. Usually, all it takes is a check-in with a close support, doing something that feels good, or taking a break. A quick visit with your therapist or doctor may also help to sort out your mood or anxiety and remind you that you have the tools to cope.

As the good days outnumber the bad ones, your fear will lessen and your confidence will rise. The fear of getting sick again does tend to stick around for a while; being prepared for these thoughts is one of the best ways to prevent them from gaining momentum. Once you've had a serious depression or anxiety problem and suffered through their devastating impact, it is understandable that you might worry that your symptoms will return. Instead of being consumed with worry, make a plan with your physician or therapist and your family about what you will do in case depression recurs. Then get on with all the other things you have to do.

Your mind-set in the early days of recovery is essential, so stay diligent, be good to yourself on difficult or negative days, and keep calling on your supports when you need them.

2. Slowly But Surely: Getting back into the Swing of Life

Women recovering from PPD or PPA and their families often wonder how much they should push themselves and if doing so will help or hinder recovery. There is no right or wrong answer to this question. The answer depends on the severity of your illness and where you are in the recovery process.

If you have had a serious depression and have been feeling well for only a few weeks, don't push yourself in the same way you would as if you had been well for several months or if you had a mild depression. When you are depressed or are beginning to get well, give yourself permission to excuse yourself from certain obligations or activities that feel particularly stressful. Stick to doing the basics at first. As your treatment progresses and you feel increasingly healthy, you can slowly reintroduce activities and responsibilities. Taking it easy when you are very ill and just beginning to recover is essential, despite what your guilty thoughts might be telling you.

You now understand how "all or nothing" thinking works and are consciously aware of it, so don't fall into these destructive ways of thinking during your recovery process. You would be surprised how many women tell me that they feel like giving up because they can't seem to do everything they used to do right away. Treat this thinking pattern like any of the other unhelpful thinking patterns: Pay attention to your thoughts, notice these patterns, and make conscious efforts to reframe your thoughts in a more realistic perspective.

Your partner or family may want you to do things that you are not ready to do. For example, they may want you to attend the family Christmas or Hanukkah party. They may tell you that it is good for you to see other people and get your mind off things. First of all, bear in mind that you know yourself best and you know where your comfort level lies. If you are in the early stages of recovery and feel that attending might be too stressful, then politely decline. If you have been feeling well for some time and think that although this event might be anxiety provoking, you would like to give it a try, go ahead. Perhaps you can attend for a short time and plan an exit strategy with your partner in advance. Let your partner and family and friends know where you are in your recovery and that you appreciate their concern, but you have to do things at your own pace.

The best strategy to getting your life back on track is to take small steps. Set your sights on achieving manageable and reasonable goals. It's okay to make mistakes when you are recovering and trying to resume your life and responsibilities with your baby, your family, and your friends. You may push it too hard sometimes when you are trying to discover your limits. You know yourself well enough to know when you have crossed a line. Assess each situation afterwards and review what worked and what didn't. Discovering your limits takes trial and error.

Take courage and pleasure from every new step you take toward health, especially in the early days when tiny steps feel as though they require Herculean strength (and let your partner know exactly what you are feeling good about so that he or she can take part in your small victories). The more steps you take, the more momentum you build. You will be surprised one day when you don't even think twice about doing things that were scary and overwhelming a short time ago while you were ill.

3. Thinking about Another Pregnancy?
Hannah was so devastated by her experience of PPA that whenever she saw a pregnant woman, she felt sorry for her. When I first met Hannah, she was adamant that she would never have another child because she did not want the gripping anxiety to recur. Hannah's PPA improved a lot with antidepressant medication and psychotherapy. As she felt better, Hannah began to see other pregnant women in a more positive way, and became less fearful of having another baby. Then, one day when her daughter was two and a half years old, Hannah called to tell me she was pregnant again—and excited!

Hannah's experience is common. For many women in the throes of their struggle with PPD or PPA, the thought of having another baby is nothing short of repulsive. They cannot imagine going through PPD or PPA again, so they conclude that the only way to avoid this is never to have another child. However, as you recover, those thoughts and doubts will diminish.

Having another baby while you are still depressed or are in the early days of recovery is not the healthiest option. Being physically and emotionally well when you decide to get pregnant and embark on the adventure all over again is ideal. Now that you are feeling good, you may also want to spend some time connecting with your baby and enjoying your life. Some people suggest that, if you have had PPD or PPA, you should wait until your first child is three or four years old before having another baby.

If you are considering another pregnancy, remember that you are now a PPD or PPA expert and have learned how to lessen its blow and limit the chances of it recurring. Just because you have had one miserable postpartum experience doesn't mean that things can't be different the next time around. You now understand the symptoms of the illness, developed a helpful treatment plan, and you can do the same thing all over again, if necessary. Read on for more information about coping with another pregnancy.

Staying Well

Once you have recovered from PPD or PPA, there are several things you can do to avoid further postpartum problems.

1. Keep It up

There is no precise time when you should stop seeking help for PPD or PPA. The best way to know is to pay attention to yourself and your feelings, consult with your professional health care providers for input, and ask your partner and close supports how they think you are doing. After talking to your therapist, if that is part of your treatment plan, ask him or her how long they think you need to remain in therapy. Keep going to your support group, if that is part of your routine, until you feel you can move on. Continue to take your medication until you can have a detailed discussion and plan with your physician. When you feel stronger, more independent, and able to take care of yourself and your baby in a safe and satisfying way, you may be able to loosen your ties to some of the extra supports. You will know when you are ready to make these changes. Make them slowly, and see how you feel with every step you take.

Of course, you need to keep eating well, exercising, and staying connected to the people you are close to. You will soon find that you naturally focus less on policing your thoughts as they become more positive and you return to your normal self. Keep checking in with yourself at least once a week. This is a wonderful way to stay connected to yourself and become more centered and comfortable than you may have ever been.

2. Get to Know Your Moods

You have learned so much about your feelings and have gotten to know yourself well throughout this process. Continue to pay attention to what triggers your bad moods or anxiety. As you notice and monitor your moods closely, you will have even more information about what makes you feel sad or happy. Then you can focus on managing the things that trigger you instead of worrying about depression and anxiety returning. Brianna recovered from PPD and was feeling really well, but had ups and downs like everyone else. She started to notice that her mood would plummet and her irritability would skyrocket

when she had no time to herself for several days in a row. Instead
of letting the depressed and irritable feelings linger for too long,
she would ask her partner and parents to help her out and give
her a break for a few hours. By identifying the triggers to her
moods, Brianna nipped the depressed feelings in the bud.

Paying attention to your moods can also help you detect
a relapse early on. This isn't common, but if you find that your
mood is consistently low and that you feel depressed again,
don't panic. You have all the tools you need to feel better, and
you understand your support network better than at any other
time in your life. You already know that it is perfectly normal
and realistic to feel down sometimes, so give yourself some
leeway and stay calm. If you find that you are slipping back into
depression, don't hesitate to resume your treatment program.
Call your doctor, talk to your partner, and get that support
network up and running. And remember that the fact that you
can recognize and address what you are experiencing means
you are already so much better.

3. Continue Getting to Know Yourself

If you are no longer experiencing depression and anxiety but
feel that there are elements of your personality that prevent
you from feeling really good or hinder your enjoyment of
your life and relationships, you may want to consider more
psychotherapy and perhaps longer-term therapy. Therapy can
continue to help you develop and grow.

Making It Easier the Next Time Around

You have survived PPD or PPA, and you may be considering
having another child. You already know that the likelihood of
recurrence is higher for women who have previously experienced PPD or PPA, but now you know all about it and how

The "W" Word: Working Outside the Home

Going back to work after having a baby is very challenging for every woman, whether or not she had PPD or PPA. Even for those women who look forward to the day they can get dressed up, stop for coffee, and drive in the car solo or take a peaceful bus ride to work, the return to work can be daunting.

Regardless of whether or not you like your job, whether or not you have to work for financial reasons, and whether or not you had PPD or PPA, going back to work after you have had a baby stirs up a mixed bag of guilt, anxiety, doubt, independence, freedom, and relief. If you have decided not to work outside the home, this can also be a complicated and emotional decision. It can be hard to know what is right for you and your family. Pursuing your career and keeping your job may be a great addition to your life, or not doing so may be a welcomed subtraction. There is no evidence that either path makes for happier, healthier children. The best decision is the one that makes for a happier, healthier mother.

Many women with PPD or PPA find that their maternity leave did not turn out as they had hoped and imagined it would because they were ill. You may have been suffering for much of the time when you were off work and only now are starting to enjoy your baby and role as a mother. If it is possible, you might welcome the opportunity to extend your maternity leave for a little while longer. This may be a great choice for you and your family.

And remember, no decision is carved in stone. You can always change your mind about whether or not to work.

to recover from it. First of all, postpartum problems may not recur. If they do, most women who experience PPD or PPA for a second time have a far easier time because there is less fear and a lot more knowledge. That means your treatment plan comes into place swiftly and efficiently. This is all good news.

1. The First Line of Defense: Get Your Support System in Order

When you get pregnant again, you and your partner can think about how you can reinstate your successful plan if PPD or PPA recurs. It is so much easier to strategize when you are healthy and optimistic than when you are depressed. You'll feel very reassured if you and your partner have a plan in place.

At the same time, take a look at your partnership before the next postpartum period and make sure it is where you want it to be. (Imagine if you had this foresight the first time around.) If your relationship is on shaky ground, work to improve it or see a couples therapist before you get pregnant or the baby arrives.

Spread the word of your pregnancy among your supports. Let them know about your pregnancy and delivery date early on so that they can be ready to support you. Anticipate the types of help and support you will need and line them up in advance. You may want to review the list for helpers in Chapter 8.

2. Reconnect with Your Mental Health Professional

If you had a psychiatrist or a therapist who helped you through your last episode of PPD or PPA, reconnect with him or her while you are thinking about getting pregnant or if you are already pregnant. Meeting and agreeing to a professional plan of action that can kick in right after you have your new baby, if necessary, is a great way for you to feel reassured, in control, and well supported. If your treatment plan worked well for you once, it can work well again.

3. Keep It Simple: Reduce the Stress in Your Life

While you are thinking about how to limit the severity of PPD or PPA, take stock of your life and lifestyle. Are there any big plans, such as changing jobs or moving homes, that you are hoping to make toward the end of your pregnancy or in the postpartum period? If the answer is yes, then stop right there. The fewer external stressors there are at a time when you will be emotionally and physically taxed, the better. Obviously, some changes are unavoidable, but try to limit the upheaval so you can go through the postpartum period on solid ground, with direct access to your established supports and personal comforts.

What a Long, Strange Trip It's Been

With great perseverance and commitment, you made it through PPD or PPA. You have worked hard to change some of your lifestyle patterns, and even harder to confront your harsh and negative thinking patterns. You found the unique treatment plan that works for you as well as professionals you trust to help and guide you. And, despite what you're accustomed to doing, you've reached out to those around you and let them know you needed their support. These are huge accomplishments. You should feel fantastic about the distance you have traveled to get to a place where you are well. There is so much strength in taking your needs and health seriously and in truly taking care of yourself. By doing so, you have given your partner, your family, and, of course, your new baby, the best reward of all—a happy, healthy you.

Acknowledgments

As I have been writing this book, I have looked forward to writing this section to express my deep thanks to all the people who helped make this book a reality. They have provided such phenomenal support, inspiration, feedback, and information. It really does take a village to write a book, particularly when you are also trying to raise two little girls, be a good partner, friend, and professional at the same time.

First, I thank my husband, true love, and partner in life, Jed. I thank you from the bottom of my heart for helping in the many ways that you did to make this book come to life, for your ever-keen wit, phenomenal loyalty, and love for me and our girls. Your support for me is unwavering.

And to my girls, Lela and Liv, thanks for being the lights of our lives.

To my mom, Susannah Dalfen. Not only are you the most supportive and encouraging mother a person could ever have, you are also an extraordinary therapist. You gave me a very early introduction to the inner workings of the human psyche and a tremendous appreciation of the value of helping others. You also provided incredibly insightful comments and feedback about this book. Without you parachuting in to help our family during the chaotic times in this writing process, we would have been lost. Thank you, for your incredible love, compassion, devotion, understanding, and strength. And to my dad, Charles Dalfen, I thank you for your love, tremendous support, and for continual excitement, aesthetic expertise, and infectious enthusiasm for this and every other project I have embarked on.

To my sister, my neighbor, and my mothering go-to-girl, Deborah Dalfen. Your support and love in every way, every day, are instrumental in my life. And thank you to Jamie Shulman for your humor, support, and encouragement, and thanks to Samantha and AJ too.

To Rachel and Jerry Schneiderman, Liz Schneiderman and Gary, Isabelle, and Emma Shub, thanks for your support.

Thanks to Susan and Judah Denburg for your love, guidance, and encouragement.

Thanks to Marijel Martinez for being so wonderful and for all of the incredible help and support that you have given to our family.

Thanks to my dear friends who have offered their professional expertise, personal input, great ideas and feedback with this project along the way. Life would not be as full or as much fun without you.

To my amazing posse of neighbors (in addition to being wonderful friends), your support in every way, from child-care help, to delicious meals, to great times, has meant the world to me.

To Dr. Bev Young, thanks for your thoughtful comments on the manuscript, and for being such a supportive and important mentor, colleague, and friend. Thanks to Dr. Eileen Sloan and the rest of the Perinatal Mental Health team for their support and input. I also thank Dr. Molyn Leszcz for your ongoing mentorship, support, and enthusiasm for this project and throughout my career. Thank you to Connie Kim for your help in preparing parts of this book.

Thanks to Ilana Valo for connecting the dots and setting the ball in motion to make this book a reality.

And, of course, a huge and ecstatic thank you goes to my editor, Leah Fairbank. Your passion, warmth, humor, and persistent encouragement were invaluable. Thanks also to Jennifer Smith, Elizabeth McCurdy, and the rest of the Wiley team for believing in this project and for helping make it happen.

And, finally, I thank all the women who have been and continue to be my patients. I have learned so much from you and have been deeply inspired by your stories and your strength. It is an honor and a privilege to be allowed into someone's inner world and I thank you for that.

Appendix:
Edinburgh Postnatal Depression Scale (EPDS)

This is the most widely used screening tool to assess PPD.

Circle the answer that comes closest to how you have felt *in the past seven days*:

1	I have been able to laugh and see the funny side of things.	As much as I always could (0) Not quite so much now (1) Definitely not so much now (2) Not at all (3)
2	I have looked forward with enjoyment to things.	As much as I ever did (0) Rather less than I used to (1) Definitely less than I used to (2) Hardly at all (3)
3	I have blamed myself unnecessarily when things went wrong.	Yes, most of the time (3) Yes, some of the time (2) Not very often (1) No, never (0)

4 I have been anxious or worried for no good reason.

No, not at all (0)
Hardly ever (1)
Yes, sometimes (2)
Yes, very often (3)

5 I have felt scared or panicky for no very good reason.

Yes, quite a lot (3)
Yes, sometimes (2)
No, not much (1)
No, not at all (0)

6 Things have been getting on top of me.

Yes, most of the time I haven't been able to cope at all (3)
Yes, sometimes I haven't been coping as well as usual (2)
No, most of the time I have coped quite well (1)
No, I have been coping as well as ever (0)

7 I have been so unhappy that I have had difficulty sleeping.

Yes, most of the time (3)
Yes, sometimes (2)
Not very often (1)
No, not at all (0)

8 I have felt sad or miserable.

Yes, most of the time (3)
Yes, quite often (2)
Not very often (1)
No, not at all (0)

9 I have been so unhappy that I have been crying.

Yes, most of the time (3)
Yes, quite often (2)
Only occasionally (1)
No, never (0)

10 The thought of harming myself has occurred to me.

Yes, quite often (3)
Sometimes (2)
Hardly ever (1)
Never (0)

Add up the numbers beside your response to each question to get your total score. If you score 10 or higher, you should contact your obstetrician, primary care provider, or a mental health professional for a more thorough evaluation. A score of 13 or more indicates that you likely have postpartum depression.

Edinburgh Postnatal Depression Scale (EPDS) J.L. Cox, J.M. Holden, R. Sagovsky, *British Journal of Psychiatry* (1987), 150, 782-786.

Programs That Specialize in Treating Women with Pregnancy and Postpartum Mental Health Issues

United States

Arizona

Women's Mental Health Program
University of Arizona
Tucson, AZ
Telephone: 520-626-3273
http://psychiatry.arizona.edu/html/programs/wmhp/overview.htm

California

Center for Neuroscience in Women's Health
Women's Wellness Clinic
Stanford University School of Medicine
Stanford, CA
Telephone: 650-736-2182
http://womensneuroscience.stanford.edu

UCLA Pregnancy and Postpartum Mood Disorders
Program
Los Angeles, CA
Telephone: 310-794-6663
http://www.semel.ucla.edu/uclamdrp/aboutPandP.html

Women's Mood Disorders Clinic
University of California at San Diego Medical Center
La Jolla, CA
Telephone: 619-543-7393
http://psychiatry.ucsd.edu

Colorado
Kempe Postpartum Depression Intervention Program
Denver, CO
Telephone: 303-864-5845
http://www.kempe.org

Connecticut
Yale Program for Women's Reproductive Behavioral Health
Department of Psychiatry
Yale University School of Medicine
New Haven, CT
Telephone: 203-764-9934
Tollfree: 1-800-Ask-Yale
(Press 2 for Yale Research Clinics, then press 1 for the WRBH)
http://info.med.yale.edu/womenshealth//impact/wrbh.html

Georgia
Emory Women's Mental Health Program
Emory University School of Medicine
Atlanta, GA
Telephone: 404-778-2524
http://www.emorywomensprogram.org

Illinois
Women's Mental Health Program
University of Illinois at Chicago
Chicago, IL
Telephone: 312-355-1223
http://www.psych.uic.edu/clinical/women.htm

Iowa
Iowa Depression and Clinical Research Center
University of Iowa Hospitals and Clinics
Iowa City, IA
Telephone: 319-335-0307, or 866-849-6636 (toll-free)
http://www.uihealthcare.com/depts/idcrc/index.html

Maryland
Women's Mood Disorders Center
The John Hopkins Hospital
Baltimore, MD
Telephone: 410-502-7449
http://www.hopkinsmedicine.org/Psychiatry/moods/clinical/clinic_
women.html

Massachusetts
MGH Center for Women's Mental Health
Massachusetts General Hospital
Boston, MA
Telephone: 617-724-2933
http://www.womensmentalhealth.org

Michigan
Women's Mental Health Program
University of Michigan
Ann Arbor, MI
Telephone: 734-764-9190
Tollfree: 800-525-5185
http://www.med.umich.edu/depression

Minnesota
Hennepin Women's Mental Health Program
Hennepin County Medical Center
Minneapolis, MN
Telephone: 612-347-3996
http://www.hcmc.org/depts/psych/mentalhealth.htm

New York
The Women's Program in the Department of Psychiatry
New York-Presbyterian Hospital
Columbia University Medical Center
Telephone: 212-305-6001
New York, NY
http://www.columbiapsychiatry.org/cs/women.html

The NYU Reproductive Psychiatry Program
New York University School of Medicine
New York, NY
Telephone: 212-263-7419
http://www.drsharilusskin.com

Payne Whitney Women's Program
Weill Cornell Medical Center
New York, NY
Telephone: 212-746-5928
http://www.cornellphysicians.com/pwwp/

Pennsylvania
Women's Behavioral HealthCARE
Western Psychiatric Institute and Clinic
Pittsburgh, PA
Telephone: 800-436-2461
http://www.womensbehavioralhealth.org

Rhode Island
Women & Infants' Hospital Day Program
Women & Infants' Hospital of Rhode Island
Providence, RI
Telephone: 401-274-1122, ext. 2870
http://womenandinfants.org

Texas
Baylor Psychiatry Clinic
Houston, TX
Telephone: 713-798-4857
http://www.bcm.edu/psychiatry/

Virginia
Virginia Commonwealth University Institute for Women's Health
Richmond, VA
Telephone: 804-560-8950 or 866-829-6626 (toll-free)
http://www.womenshealth.vcu.edu

Washington, DC
Women's Mental Health
Georgetown University Hospital
Washington, DC
Telephone: 202-687-8609
http://www.georgetownuniversityhospital.org

Canada

British Columbia
The British Columbia Reproductive Mental Health Program
Vancouver, BC
Telephone: 604-875-3060 or 604-875-2025
http://bcwomens.ca

Ontario
Perinatal Mental Health Program
Mount Sinai Hospital
Toronto, ON
Telephone: 416-586-4800, ext. 8419
http://www.mountsinai.on.ca/care/psych/patient-programs/maternal-infant-perinatal-psychiatry

Reproductive Life Stages Program
Women's College Hospital
Toronto, ON
Telephone: 416-323-6400, ext. 5635
http://womenscollegehospital.ca/health/index.html

Women's Mental Health Clinic
Toronto General Hospital
Toronto, ON
Telephone: 416-340-3048
http://www.uhn.ca/clinics_&_services/clinics/womens_mental_health.asp

Ottawa Regional Perinatal Mental Health Program
The Ottawa Hospital—General Campus
Ottawa, ON
Telephone: 613-737-8010

Women's Health Concerns Clinic
St. Joseph's Healthcare Hamilton
Hamilton, ON
Telephone: 905-522-1155, ext. 33031
http://www.stjoes.ca

Nova Scotia
Reproductive Mental Health Service
IWK Health Centre
Department of Psychiatry
Dalhousie University
Halifax, NS
Phone; 902-470-8098
Fax:902-470-6760

Resources

General Pregnancy and Postpartum

Recommended Reading

The Mother of All Pregnancy Books: An All-Canadian Guide to Conception, Birth, and Everything in Between by Ann Douglas, John Wiley & Sons Canada, Ltd., 2000.

The Girlfriends' Guide to Pregnancy: Or Everything Your Doctor Won't Tell You by Vicki Iovine, Simon & Schuster, 1995.

What to Expect When You're Expecting by Heidi Murkoff, Workman Publishing Company; 3rd edition, 2002.

The New Mom's Survival Guide: How to reclaim your body, your health, your sanity, and your sex life after having a baby by Jennifer Wider M.D., Random House, Bantam, 2008.

Resources

American College of Obstetricians and Gynecologists (ACOG)
http://www.acog.com

Baby Center
http://www.babycenter.com

Canadian Medical Association
http://www.cma.ca

National Women's Health Information Center, a Project of the US
Department of Health and Human Services, Office on Women's Health
http://www.4woman.gov/faw/postpartum.htm

The Society of Obstetricians and Gynecologists of Canada
http://ww.sogc.org

General Mental Health
Recommended Reading
The Feeling Good Handbook by David Burns, Plume, 1999.

Mind over Mood: Change How You Feel by Changing the Way You Think by
Dennis Greenberger and Christine Padersky, Guildford Press, 1995.

An Unquiet Mind: A Memoir of Moods and Madness by Ken R. Jamison,
Vintage, 1997.

My Depression: A Picture Book by Elizabeth Swados, Hyperion Books,
2005.

Resources
United States
American Psychiatric Association
http://www.psych.org

American Psychological Association
http://www.apa.org

Anxiety Disorders Association of America (ADAA)
http://www.adaa.org

Depression and Bipolar Support Alliance
http://www.dbsalliance.org

National Alliance on Mental Illness
http://www.nami.org

National Institute of Mental Health
http://nimh.nih.gov

National Mental Health Association
http://nmha.org

National Mental Health Information Center
http://www.mentalhealth.org

Canada

Canadian Association of Social Workers
http://www.casw.acts.ca

Canadian Mental Health Association
http://www.cmha.ca

Canadian Network for Mood and Anxiety Treatment
http://canmat.org

Canadian Psychiatric Association
http://www.cpa-apc.org

Canadian Psychological Association
http://www.cpa.ca

Centre for Addiction and Mental Health
http://www.camh.net

Mood Disorders Association of Ontario
http://checkupfromtheneckup.ca

Postpartum and Pregnancy-Related Mental Health Problems

Recommended Reading

She's Had a Baby: And I'm Having a Meltdown by James D. Barron, Harper Paperbacks, 1999.

Postpartum Mood and Anxiety Disorders by Cheryl Beck and Jeanne Driscoll, *A Guide.* Jones & Bartlett Publishers, 2005.

Beyond the Blues: A Guide to Understanding and Treating Prenatal and Postpartum Depression by Shoshana S. Bennett and Pec Indman, Moodswings Press, 2003.

The Postpartum Husband: Practical Solutions for Living with Postpartum Depression by Karen Kleiman, Xlibris, 2001.

What Am I Thinking? Having a Baby after Postpartum Depression by Karen Kleiman, Xlibris, 2005.

This Isn't What I Expected: Overcoming Postpartum Depression by Karen Kleiman and Valerie D Raskin, Bantam Books, 1994.

Pregnancy Blues: What Every Woman Needs to Know about Depression during Pregnancy by Shaila Kulkarni Misri, Random House, 2005.

Shouldn't I Be Happy?: Emotional Problems of Pregnant and Postpartum Women by Shaila Kulkarni Misri, Free Press, 2002.

A Deeper Shade of Blue: A Woman's Guide to Recognizing and Treating Depression in Her Childbearing Years by Ruta Nonacs, Simon & Schuster, 2006.

Behind the Smile: My Journey out of Postpartum Depression by Marie Osmond, Warner Books, 2001.

The Mother-to-Mother Postpartum Depression Support Book: Real Stories from Women Who Lived through It and Recovered by Sandra Poulin, Penguin Group, 2006.

Understanding Your Moods When You're Expecting: Emotions, Mental Health, and Happiness—before, during, and after Pregnancy by Lucy J. Puryear, Houghton Mifflin Company, 2007.

Down Came the Rain: My Journey through Postpartum Depression by Brooke Shields Hyperion, 2005.

Women's Moods: What Every Woman Must Know about Hormones, the Brain, and Emotional Health by Deborah Sichel and Jeanne Watson Driscoll, Harper Paperbacks, 2000.

Postpartum Depression Demystified: An Essential Guide to Understanding and Overcoming the Most Common Complication after Childbirth by Joyce A Venis and Suzanne McCloskey, Marlowe and Company, 2007.

Resources

Academy of Breastfeeding Medicine
http://www.bfmed.org

Best Start
http://www.beststart.org
http://www.lifewithnewbaby.ca

Breastfeeding and Medication Information
http://neonatal.ttuhsc.edu/lact/index.html

Centre for Addiction and Mental Health—Postpartum Depression: A
Guide for Front-line Health and Social Services Providers
http://www.camh.net/publications/camh_publications/postpartum_
depression_guide.html

Depression during Breastfeeding
http://www.pregnancyanddepresion.com/breastfeeding.html

Emory University Women's Mental Health Program
http://www.emorywomensprogram.org

Health Resources and Service Administration: Depression during and
after Pregnancy: A Resource for Women, Their Families, and Friends
http://www.mchb.hrsa.gov/pregnancyandbeyond/depression

The Marcé Society
http://www.marcesociety.com

MGH Center for Women's Mental Health
http://www.womensmentalhealth.org

Motherisk
http://www.motherisk.org/breastfeeding/index.php3

North American Society for Psychosocial OB/GYN
http://www.naspog.org

Our Sister's Place
http://www.oursistersplace.ca

The Pacific Post Partum Support Society
http://www.postpartum.org

Postpartum Progress (blog)
http://postpartumprogress.typepad.com/weblog

Postpartum Support International
http://www.postpartum.net

Reprotox
http://www.reprotox.org

Women's Health Matters—Baby Blues or Postpartum Depression?
http://www.womenshealthmatters.ca/facts/quick_show_d.
cfm?number=480

Support for Partners
Dads Adventure
http://www.newdads.com

The National Center for Fathering
http://www.fathers.com

Postpartum Dads
http://www.postpartumdads.org

Baby Care and Parenting Resources
Recommended Reading
The Mother of All Baby Books: an all-Canadian guide to baby's first year by
Ann Douglas, John Wiley & Sons Canada Ltd., 2001.

The Baby Whisperer by Tracy Hogg, Ballantine Books, 2005.

The Happiest Baby on the Block by Harvey Karp, Bantam Dell, 2003.

Your Baby and Child: From Birth to Age Five by Penelope Leach Alfred A.
Knopf Inc., 2000.

*Gentle Baby Care: No-Cry, No-Fuss, No-Worry—Essential Tips for Raising
Your Baby* by Elizabeth Pantely, McGraw-Hill, 2004.

The No-Cry Sleep Solution: Gentle Ways to Help Your Baby Sleep through the Night by Elizabeth Pantely, McGraw-Hill, 2002.

Breaking the Good Mom Myth: Every Mom's Modern Guide to Getting Past Perfection, Regaining Sanity, and Raising Great Kids by Alyson Schafer, John Wiley & Sons Canada Ltd., 2007.

Healthy Sleep Habits, Happy Child by Marc Weissbluth, Random House, 2005.

Resources

Babycenter
http://www.babycenter.com

Canadian Health Network
http://www.canadian-health-nework.ca

Canadian Pediatrics Society
http://www.cpa.ca

Children's Mental Health Resources
http://www.aacap.org

Kids' Health
http://kidshealth.org

Relationship Issues

Recommended Reading

And Baby Makes Three: The Six-Step Plan for Preserving Marital Intimacy and Rekindling Romance after Baby Arrives by John M. Gottman and Julie Schwartz Gottman, Random House, 2007.

Gottman, John M. and Nan Silver. *The Seven Principles for Making Marriage Work* by John M. Gottman and Nan Silver, Three Rivers Press, 1999.

Getting the Love You Want: A Guide for Couples, 20th Anniversary Edition by Harville Hendrix, Henry Holt and Company, 2007.

The Big Picture
Making Large Scale Change

We have talked a lot about individual and family approaches to treating PPD and PPA. There are some political and legislative changes that are helping to address PPD and to reduce the incidence of it. Most of the political headway on PPD has been made in the United States.

The State of New Jersey introduced a law in April 2006, which is known as the Postpartum Depression Law. This law is the first of its kind and the most comprehensive PPD law in the United States. It mandates all health care providers to screen new mothers for PPD prior to their discharge from the hospital, after delivery, as well as at their postpartum follow-up visits. It also requires health care facilities and health care providers to educate and inform new mothers and their families about PPD. California, Texas, Washington, and New York State have also enacted state legislation related to PPD, mostly to increase information for new moms and public awareness.

On a national level, in 2003, the Melanie Blocker Stokes Postpartum Depression Research and Care Act was introduced by US Congressman Bobby Rush (D-IL). Melanie Blocker Stokes committed suicide while she suffered from postpartum psychosis. The Act called for improving services for women suffering from PPD and postpartum psychosis as well as for increasing US federal funding for research and service delivery for these illnesses. This was passed in the U.S. House of Representatives in October 2007.

In 2006, US senators Robert Menendez (D-NJ) and Richard Durbin (D-IL) introduced The MOTHERS Act (Mom's Opportunity to Access Help, Education, Research, and Support for Postpartum Depression Act) to the Senate. This Act incorporated The Melanie Blocker Stokes Act. It proposes to increase education and screening for new mothers and increase funding for research into postpartum mental illness. It also proposes to help health care providers improve services for those suffering from PPD. The Melanie Blocker Stokes MOTHERS Act has yet to be passed by the US Senate into legislation.

These legislative and political initiatives can do a lot for postpartum mental illness. They are an important way to increase public awareness and reduce stigma. New funding will support research that will improve our understanding of postpartum illnesses and our capacity to treat the many women who suffer. Legal and political action can also create significant changes to national and local health care systems that will help prevent PPD and improve the treatment of this common and devastating illness.

Bibliography

Abramowitz, J. S., Schwartz, S. A., Moore, K. M. et al. (2003). Obsessive-compulsive symptoms in pregnancy and the puerperium: A review of the literature. *Journal of Anxiety Disorders*, 17 (4), 461–478.

Abrams, S. M., Field, T., Scafidi, F. et al. (1995). Newborns of depressed mothers. *Infant Mental Health Journal*, 16 (3), 233–239.

The Academy of Breastfeeding Medicine Protocol Committee. (2008). ABM clinical protocol #18: Use of antidepressants in nursing mothers. *Breastfeeding Medicine*, 3 (1), 44–52.

Addis, A. & Koren, G. (2000). Safety of fluoxetine during the first trimester of pregnancy: A meta-analytical review of epidemiological studies. *Psychological Medicine*, 30 (1), 89–94.

Akman, C., Uguz, F. & Kaya, N. (2007). Postpartum-onset major depression is associated with personality disorders. *Comprehensive Psychiatry*, 48, 343–347.

Alpert, J. E., Papakostas, G., Mischoulon, D. et al. (2004). S-adenosyl-L-methionine (SAMe) as an adjunct for resistant major depressive disorder: An open trial following partial or nonresponse to selective serotonin reuptake inhibitors or venlafaxine. *Journal of Clinical Psychopharmacology*, 24 (6), 661–664.

Altshuler, L., Cohen, L., Moline, M. et al. (2001). Expert consensus guideline series: Treatment of depression in women. *Postgraduate Medicine Special Report*, 1–116.

Altshuler, L., Cohen, L. S., Szuba, M. P. et al. (1996). Pharmacologic management of psychiatric illness in pregnancy: Dilemmas and guidelines. *American Journal of Psychiatry*, 153, 592–606.

Alwan, S., Reefhuis, J., Rasmussen, S. A. et al. (2007). Use of selective serotonin-reuptake inhibitors in pregnancy and the risk of birth defects. *New England Journal of Medicine*, 356 (26), 2684–2692.

American Family Physician. (2005). *Insomnia: How to get a good night's sleep*. http://www.aafp.org/afp/20051001/1309ph.html.

American Psychological Association. (2004). *How to find help through psychotherapy*. http://www.apa.org.

Amin, Z., Canli, T. & Epperson, C. N. (2005). Effect of estrogen-serotonin interactions on mood and cognition. *Behavioral & Cognitive Neuroscience Reviews*, 4 (1), 43–58.

Andersson, L., Sundstrom-Poromaa, I., Bixo, M. et al. (2003). Point prevalence of psychiatric disorders during the second trimester of pregnancy: A population-based study. *American Journal of Obstetrics & Gynecology*, 189 (1), 148–154.

Andersson, L., Sundstrom-Poromaa, I., Wulff, M. et al. (2004). Neonatal outcome following maternal antenatal depression and anxiety: A population-based study. *American Journal of Epidemiology*, 159 (9), 872–881.

Appleby, L. Warner, R., Whitton, A. et al. (1997). A controlled study of fluoxetine and cognitive-behavioral counseling in the treatment of postnatal depression. *British Medical Journal*, 314 (7085), 932–936.

Armstrong, D. S. (2004). Impact of prior perinatal loss on subsequent pregnancies. *Journal of Obstetric, Gynecologic & Neonatal Nursing*, 33 (6), 765–773.

Austin, M. P., Hadzi-Pavlovic, D., Leader, L. et al. (2005). Maternal trait anxiety, depression, and life event stress in pregnancy: Relationships with infant temperament. *Early Human Development*, 81 (2), 183–190.

Beck, C. (1996). A meta-analysis of predictors of postpartum depression. *Nursing Research*, 45 (5), 297–303.

Beck, C. T. (2001). Predictors of postpartum depression: An update. *Nursing Research*, 50(5), 275–285.

Bennett, Shoshana S. & Indman, P. (2003). *Beyond the blues: A guide to understanding and treating prenatal and postpartum depression.* San Jose: Moodswings Press.

Blackmore, E. R. et al. (2006). Obstetric variables associated with bipolar affective puerperal psychosis. *British Journal of Psychiatry,* 188, 32-36.

Bonari, L., Pinto, N., Ahn, E. et al. (2004). Perinatal risks of untreated depression during pregnancy. *Canadian Journal of Psychiatry,* 49 (11), 726-735.

Bowlby, J. (1990). *Secure base: Parent-child attachment and healthy human development.* New York: Basic Books.

Brown, G. W., Harris, T. O. & Hepworth, C. (1995). Loss, humiliation, and entrapment among women developing depression: A patient and non-patient comparison. *Psychological Medicine,* 25 (1), 7-21.

Brown, G. W. & Moran, P. M. (1997). Single mothers, poverty, and depression. *Psychological Medicine,* 27 (1), 21-33.

Brunton, P. J. & Russell, J. A. (2008). The expectant brain: Adapting for motherhood. *Neuroscience,* 9, 11-25.

Burns, D. D. (1999). *The feeling good handbook.* New York: Plume.

Burt, V. K., Suri, R., Altshuler, L. et al. (2001). The use of psychotropic medications during breastfeeding. *American Journal of Psychiatry,* 158, 1001-1009.

Casper, R. C. et al. (2003), Follow-up of children of depressed mothers exposed or not exposed to antidepressant drugs during pregnancy. *Journal of Pediatrics,* 142, 402-408.

Chabrol, H., Teissedre, F., Saint-Jean, M. et al. (2002). Prevention and treatment of post-partum depression: A controlled randomized study on women at risk. *Psychological Medicine,* 32 (6), 1039-1047.

Chambers, C. D, Hernandez-Diaz, S., Van Marter, L. J. et al. (2006) Selective-serotonin reuptake inhibitors and risk of persistent pulmonary hypertension of the newborn. *New England Journal of Medicine,* 354 (6), 579-587.

Chambers, C. D., Johnson, K., Dick, L. et al. (1996). Birth outcomes in pregnant women taking fluoxetine. *New England Journal of Medicine,* 335 (14), 1010-1015.

Chaudron, L. H. & Jefferson, J. W. (2000). Mood stabilizers during breastfeeding: A review. *Journal of Clinical Psychiatry,* 61 (2), 79-90.

Chaudron, L. H. & Pies, R. W. (2003). The relationship between postpartum psychosis and bipolar disorder: A review. *Journal of Clinical Psychiatry,* 64 (11), 1284-1292.

Chaudron, L. H. & Schoenecker, C. J. (2004). Bupropion and breast-feeding: A case of a possible infant seizure. *Journal of Clinical Psychiatry*, 65, 881-882.

Cohen, L. S., Altshuler, L. L., Harlow, B. L. et al. (2006). Relapse of major depression during pregnancy in women who maintain or discontinue antidepressant treatment. *Journal of the American Medical Association*, 295, 499-507.

Cohen, L. S., Friedman, J. M., Jefferson, J. W. et al. (1994). A reevaluation of risk of in utero exposure to lithium. *JAMA*, 271 (2), 146-150.

Cohen, L. S., Heller, V. L., Bailer, J. W. et al. (2004). Birth outcomes following prenatal exposure to fluoxetine. *Biological Psychiatry*, 48 (1), 996-1000.

Cohen, L. S., Nonacs, R. M., Bailey, J. W. et al. (2004). Relapse of depression during pregnancy following antidepressant discontinuation: A preliminary prospective study. *Archives of Women's Mental Health*, 7 (4), 217-221.

Cohen, L. S., Sichel, D. A., Robertson, L. M. et al. (1995). Postpartum prophylaxis for women with bipolar disorder. *American Journal of Psychiatry*, 152 (11), 164-165.

Cohen, L. S., Viguera, A. C., Bouffard, S. M. et al. (2001). Venlafaxine in the treatment of postpartum depression. *Journal of Clinical Psychiatry*, 62 (8), 592-596.

Collins, N. L., Dunkel-Schetter, C., Lobel, M. et al. (1993). Social support in pregnancy: Psychosocial correlates of birth outcomes and postpartum depression. *Journal of Personality and Social Psychology*, 65 (6), 1243-1258.

Conover, E. A. (2002). Over-the-counter products: Nonprescription medications, nutraceuticals, and herbal agents. *Clinical Obstetrics & Gynecology*, 45 (1), 89-98.

Correia, L. L. & Martins Linhares, M. B. (2007). Maternal anxiety in the pre- and postnatal period: A literature review. *Rev Latino-am Enfermagem*, 15 (4), 677-683.

Cowan, C. & Cowan, P. (1992). *When parents become partners: The big life change for couples.* New York: Basic Books.

Cox, J. L., Holden, J. M. & Sagovsky, R. (1987). Detection of postnatal depression: Development of the 10-item Edinburgh Postnatal Depression Scale. *British Journal of Psychiatry*, 150, 782-786.

Daley, A. J., MacArthur, C. & Winter, H. (2007). The role of exercise in treating postpartum depression: A review of the literature. *Journal of Midwifery and Women's Health*, 52, 56-62.

Davis, E. P., Glynn, L. M., Schetter, C. D. et al. (2007). Prenatal exposure to maternal depression and cortisol influences infant temperament. *Journal of the American Academy of Child & Adolescent Psychiatry*, 46 (6), 737–746.

Dennis, C.-L. (2003). The effect of peer support on postpartum depression: A pilot randomized and controlled trial. *Canadian Journal of Psychiatry*, 48 (2), 115–124.

Dennis, C.-L. (2004). Treatment of postpartum depression, part 2: A critical review of nonbiological interventions. *Journal of Clinical Psychiatry*, 65 (9), 1252–1265.

Dennis, C.-L. & Hodnett, E. (2008). Psychosocial and psychological interventions for treating postpartum depression (review). *Cochrane Database of Systematic Reviews*, 4, Art. No.: CD006116.

Dennis, C.-L. & McQueen, K. (2007). Does maternal postpartum depressive symptomatology influence infant feeding outcomes? *Acta Paediatrica*, 96, 590–594.

Dennis, C.-L. & Ross, L. (2005). Relationships among infant sleep patterns, maternal fatigue, and development of depressive symptomatology. *Birth*, 32 (3), 187–193.

Dennis, C.-L. & Ross, L. E. (2006). Depressive symptomatology in the immediate postnatal period:

Identifying maternal characteristics related to true- and false-positive screening scores. *The Canadian Journal of Psychiatry*, 51 (5), 265–273.

Dennis, C.-L. & Ross, L. (2006). Women's perceptions of partner support and conflict in the development of postpartum depressive symptoms. *Journal of Advanced Nursing*, 56 (6), 588–599.

Dennis, C.-L. & Stewart, D. E. (2004). Treatment of postpartum depression, part 1: A critical review of biological interventions. *Journal of Clinical Psychiatry*, 65, 1242–1251.

De Smet, P. A. (2002). Herbal remedies. *New England Journal of Medicine*, 347 (25), 2046–2056.

De Smet, P. A. (2004). Health risks of herbal remedies: An update. *Clinical Pharmacology & Therapeutics*, 76 (1), 1–17.

Dietz, P. M. et al. (2007). Clinically identified maternal depression before, during, and after pregnancies ending in live births. *American Journal of Psychiatry*, 164, 1515.

Edinger, J. D., Wohlgemuth, W. K., Radtke, R. A. et al. (2001). Cognitive behavioural therapy for treatment of chronic primary insomnia: A randomized controlled trial. *Journal of the American Medical Association*, 285 (14), 1856–1864.

Einarson, A., Bonari, L., Voyer-Lavigne, S. et al. (2003). A multi-centre prospective controlled study to determine the safety of tra-zodone and nefazodone use during pregnancy. *Canadian Journal of Psychiatry*, 48 (2), 106-110.

Einarson, T. R. & Einarson, A. (2005). Newer antidepressants in pregnancy and rates of major malformations: A meta-analysis of prospective comparative studies. *Pharmacoepidemiology and Drug Safety*, 14 (12), 823-827.

Einarson, A., Pistelli, A., DeSantis, M. et al. (2008). Evaluation of the risk of congenital cardiovascular defects associated with use of parox-etine during pregnancy. *American Journal of Psychiatry*, 165: 749-752

Einarson, A., Sarkar, M., Lavigne, S. V. et al. (2001). Pregnancy out-come following gestational expo-sure to venlafaxine: A multicenter prospective controlled study. *American Journal of Psychiatry*, 158 (10), 1728-1730.

Ernst, C. L. & Goldberg, J. F. (2002). The reproductive safety profile of mood stabilizers, atypical antipsychotics, and broad-spec-trum psychotropics. *Journal of Clinical Psychiatry*, 4, 42-55.

Evans, J., Heron, J., Francomb, H. et al. (2001). Cohort study of depressed mood during pregnancy and after childbirth. *British Medical Journal*, 323 (7307), 257-260.

Everingham, C. R., Heading, G. H. & Connor, L. (2006). Couples' experiences of postnatal depres-sion: A framing analysis of cultural identity, gender, and communica-tion. *Social Science & Medicine*, 62, 1745-1756.

Field, T., Hernandez-Reif, M. & Feijo, L. (2002). Breastfeeding in depressed mother-infant dyads. *Early Child Development and Care*, 172 (6), 539-545.

Fleming, A. S., Klein, E. & Corter, C. (1992). The effects of a social sup-port group on depression, maternal attitudes, and behavior in new mothers. *Journal of Child Psychology and Psychiatry*, 33 (4), 685-698.

Fochtmann, L. J. & Gelenberg, A. J. (2005). *Guideline watch: Practice guideline for the treatment of pa-tients with major depressive disor-der* (2nd ed.). Arlington: American Psychiatric Association.

Forray, A. & Ostroff, R. B. (2007) The use of electroconvulsive therapy in postpartum affective disorders. *Journal of ECT*, 23 (3), 188-193.

Fossey, L., Papiernik, E. & Byd-lowski, M. (1997). Postpartum blues: A clinical syndrome and predictor of postnatal depression. *Journal of Psychosomatic Obstetrics & Gynecology*, 18 (1), 17-21.

Fraiberg, S. (1975). Ghosts in the nursery: A psychoanalytic approach to the problem of impaired infant-mother relationships. *Journal of the American Academy of Child and Adolescent Psychiatry*, 14 (3), 387-421.

Freeman, M. P. (2006). Omega-3 fatty acids and perinatal depression: A review of the literature and recommendations for future research. *Prostaglandins Leukot Essential Fatty Acids*, 75 (4-5), 291-297.

Freeman, M. P. (2007). Antenatal depression: Navigating the treatment dilemmas. *American Journal of Psychiatry*, 164, 1162-1165.

Freeman, M. P., Davis, M., Sniha, P. et al. (2008). Omega-3 fatty acids and supportive psychotherapy for perinatal depression: A randomized placebo-controlled study. *Journal of Affective Disorders*, 110 (1-2), 142-148.

Freeman, M. P., Helgason, C. & Hill, R. A. (2004). Selected integrative medicine treatments for depression: Considerations for women. *Journal of the American Medical Women's Association*, 59 (3), 216-224.

Gabbard, G. O. (2007). Psychotherapy in psychiatry. *International Review of Psychiatry*, 19 (1), 5-12.

Gandhi, S. G. et al. (2006). Maternal and neonatal outcomes after attempted suicide. *Obstetrics & Gynecology*, 107, 984-990.

Gaster, B. & Holroyd, J. (2000). St. John's wort for depression: A systematic review. *Archives of Internal Medicine*, 160 (2), 152-156.

Geddes, J. R., Carney, S. M., Davies, C. et al. (2003). Relapse prevention with antidepressant drug treatment in depressive disorders: A systematic review. *Lancet*, 361 (9358), 653-661.

Gentile, S. (2004) Clinical utilization of atypical antipsychotics in pregnancy and lactation. *Annals of Pharmacotherapy*, 38 (7-8), 1265-1271.

Gentile, S. (2008) Infant safety with antipsychotic therapy in breastfeeding: A systematic review. *Journal of Clinical Psychiatry*, 69 (4), 666-673.

George, L. K., Blazer, D. G., Hughes, D. C. et al. (1989). Social support and the outcome of major depression. *British Journal of Psychiatry*, 154, 478-485.

Goldstein, D. J. (1995). Effects of third trimester fluoxetine exposure on the newborn. *Clinical Psychopharmacology*, 15, 417-420.

Goldstein, D. J. & Fung, M. C. (2000). Olanzapine-exposed pregnancies and lactation: Early experience. *Journal of Clinical Psychopharmacology*, 20, 399-403.

Goldstein, D. J., Sundell, K. L. & Corbin, L. A. (1997). Birth outcomes in pregnant women taking fluoxetine. *New England Journal of Medicine*, 336 (12), 872-873.

Gottman, J. M. (1993). The roles of conflict engagement, escalation, and avoidance in marital interaction: A longitudinal view of five types of couples. *Journal of Consulting & Clinical Psychology*, 61 (1), 6-15.

Gottman, J. M. & Schwartz Gottman, J. (2007). *And baby makes three: The six-step plan for preserving marital intimacy and rekindling romance after baby arrives*. New York: Random House.

Greene, M. F. (2007). Teratogenicity of SSRIs—Serious concern or much ado about little? *New England Journal of Medicine*, 356 (26), 2732-2733.

Greenberger, D. & Padesky, C. (1995). *Mind over mood: Change how you feel by changing the way you think*. New York: The Guildford Press.

Grigoriadis, S. & Ravitz, P. (2007). An approach to interpersonal psychotherapy for postpartum depression: Focusing on interpersonal changes. *Canadian Family Physician*, 53 (9), 1469-1475.

Halberg, P. et al. (2005). The use of selective serotonin reuptake inhibitors during pregnancy and breastfeeding: A review and clinical aspects. *Journal of Clinical Psychopharmacology*, 25, 59-73.

Halbreich, U. (2004). Prevalence of mood symptoms and depressions during pregnancy: Implications for clinical practice and research. *CNS Spectrums*, 9 (3), 177-184.

Harlow, B. L., Vitonis, A. F., Sparen, P. et al. (2007). Incidence of hospitalization for postpartum psychotic and bipolar episodes in women with and without prior pregnancy or prenatal psychiatric hospitalizations. *Archives of General Psychiatry*, 64 (1), 42-48.

Hart, S., Field, T. & Roitfarb, M. (1999). Depressed mothers' assessments of their neonates' behaviors. *Infant Mental Health Journal*, 20 (2), 200-210.

Hatton, D. C., Harrison-Hohner, J., Matarazzo, J. et al. (2007). Missed antenatal depression among high-risk women: A secondary analysis. *Archives of Women's Mental Health*, 10 (3), 121-123.

Hay, D. F., Pawlby, S., Sharp, D. et al. (2001). Intellectual problems shown by 11-year-old children whose mothers had postnatal depression. *Journal of Child Psychology and Psychiatry*, 42 (7), 871-889.

Hemels, M. E., Einarson, A., Koren, G. et al. (2005). Antidepressant use during pregnancy and the rates of spontaneous abortions: A meta-analysis. *Annals of Pharma-cotherapy*, 39 (5), 803-809.

Henderson, J. J., Evans, S. F., Straton, J. A. et al. (2003). Impact of postnatal depression on breastfeeding duration. *Birth*, 30 (3), 175-180.

Hendrick, V., Altshuler, L., Strouse, T. et al. (2000). Postpartum and nonpostpartum depression: Differences in presentation and response to pharmacologic treatment. *Depression & Anxiety*, 11 (2), 66-72.

Hendrick, V., Altshuler, L. & Suri, R. (1998). Hormonal changes in the postpartum and implications for postpartum depression. *Psychosomatics*, 39, 93-101.

Hendrick, V., Fukuchi, A., Altshuler, L. et al. (2003). Use of sertraline, paroxetine, and fluvoxamine by nursing women. *British Journal of Psychiatry*, 179, 163-166.

Hendrick, V., Smith, L. M., Suri, R. et al. (2003). Birth outcomes after prenatal exposure to antidepressant medication. *American Journal of Obstetrics and Gynecology*, 188 (3), 812-815.

Hendrick, V., Stowe, Z. N., Altshuler, L. et al. (2000). Paroxetine use during breastfeeding. *Journal of Clinical Psychopharmacology*, 20 (5), 587-589.

Hendrick, V., Stowe, Z. N., Altshuler, L. et al. (2001). Fluoxetine

and norfluoxetine concentrations in nursing infants and breast milk. *Biological Psychiatry*, 50 (1), 775-782.

Henshaw, C. (2003). Mood disturbance in the early puerperium: A review. *Archives of Women's Mental Health*, 6 (suppl. 2), S33-S42.

Henshaw, C., Foreman, D. & Cox, J. (2004). Postnatal blues: A risk factor for postnatal depression. *Journal of Psychosomatic Obstetrics & Gynecology*, 24 (3-4), 267-272.

Heron, J., O'Connor, T. G., Evans, J. et al. (2004). The course of anxiety and depression through pregnancy and the postpartum in a community sample. *Journal of Affective Disorders*, 80 (1), 65-73.

Hiscock, H., Bayer, J., Gold, L. et al. (2007). Improving infant sleep and maternal mental health: A cluster randomized trial. *Archives of Disease in Childhood*, 92, 952-958.

Hiscock, H. & Wake, M. (2001) Infant sleep problems and postnatal depression: A community-based study. *Pediatrics*, 107 (6), 13171322.

Holmes, L. B. (2002). The teratogenicity of anticonvulsant drugs: A progress report. *Journal of Medical Genetics*, 39 (4), 245-247.

Hostetter, A., Ritchie, J. C. & Stowe, Z. N. (2000). Amniotic fluid and umbilical cord blood concentrations of antidepressants in three women. *Biological Psychiatry*, 48 (10), 1032–1034.

Iqbal, M. M., Sobhan, T. & Ryals, T. (2002). Effects of commonly used benzodiazepines on the fetus, the neonate, and the nursing infant. *Psychiatric Services*, 53 (1), 39–49.

Jindal, R. D. & Thase, M. E. (2003). Integrating psychotherapy and pharmacotherapy to improve outcomes among patients with mood disorders. *Psychiatric Services*, 54 (11), 1484–1490.

Joffe, H. & Cohen, L. (1998). Estrogen, serotonin, and mood disturbances: Where is the therapeutic bridge? *Biological Psychiatry*, 44, 798–811.

Kendall, R. E., Chalmers, J. C. & Platz, C. (1987). Epidemiology of puerperal psychoses. *British Journal of Psychiatry*, 150, 662–673.

Kendall-Tackett, K. (2007) A new paradigm for depression in new mothers: The central role of inflammation and how breastfeeding and anti-inflammatory treatments protect maternal mental health. *International Breastfeeding Journal*, 2 (6),

Kennedy, S. H., Lam, R. W. & the CANMAT Depression Working Group. (2001). Clinical guidelines for the treatment of depressive disorders. *Canadian Journal of Psychiatry*, 46 (suppl. 1), 1S–92S.

Kleiman, K. (2001). *The postpartum husband: Practical solutions for living with postpartum depression*. Philadelphia: Xlibris.

Kleiman, K. (2005). *What am I thinking? Having a baby after postpartum depression*. Philadelphia: Xlibris.

Kleiman, K. R. & Raskin, V. D. (1994). *This isn't what I expected: Overcoming postpartum depression*. New York: Bantam Books.

Klerman, G. L., Weissman, M. M., Rounsaville, B. J. et al. (1984). *Interpersonal psychotherapy of depression*. New York: Basic Books.

Klier, C. M., Geller, P. A. & Neugebauer, R. (2000). Minor depressive disorder in the context of a miscarriage. *Journal of Affective Disorders*, 59 (1), 13–21.

Klier, C. M., Schafter, M. R., Schmid-Siegel, B. et al. (2002). St. John's wort (*Hypericum perforate*): Is it safe during breastfeeding? *Pharmacopsychiatry*, 35 (1), 29–30.

Knekt, P., Kindfors, O., Harkanen, T. et al. (2007). Randomized trial on the effectiveness of long- and short-term psychodynamic psychotherapy and solution-focused therapy on psychiatric symptoms during a 3-year follow-up. *Psychological Medicine*, 16, 1-15.

Kramer, M. S., Fombonne, E., Igumnov, S. et al. (2008). Effects of prolonged and exclusive breast-feeding on child behavior and maternal adjustment: Evidence from a large, randomized trial. *Pediatrics*, 121 (3), 435-440.

Kupfer, D., Frank, E., Perel, J. et al. (1992) Five-year outcome for maintenance therapies in recurrent depression. *Archives of General Psychiatry*, 49 (10), 769-773.

Lawrence, E., Nylen, K. & Cobb, R. J. (2007). Prenatal expectations and marital satisfaction over the transition to parenthood. *Journal of Family Psychology*, 21 (2), 155-164.

Lee, A., Minhas, R., Matsuda, N., Lam, M. et al. (2003). The safety of St. John's wort (*Hypericum perforatum*) during breastfeeding. *Journal of Clinical Psychiatry*, 64 (8), 966-968.

Lee, A. M., Lam, S. K., Sze, M. L. et al. (2007). Prevalence, course, and risk factors for antenatal anxiety and depression. *Obstetrics & Gynecology*, 110 (5), 1102-1112.

Letters to the Editor. (2007). Mirtazapine and breastfeeding: Maternal and infant plasma levels. *American Journal of Psychiatry*, 164 (2), 348-349.

Linde, K., Berner, M., Egger, M. et al. (2005). St. John's wort for depression: Meta-analysis of randomized controlled trials. *British Journal of Psychiatry*, 186, 99-107.

Logsdon, M. C., McBride, A. B. & Birkimer, J. C. (1994). Social support and postpartum depression. *Research in Nursing Health*, 17, 449-457.

Louik, C., Lin, A. E., Werler, M. M. et al. (2007). First-trimester use of selective serotonin-reuptake inhibitors and the risk of birth defects. *New England Journal of Medicine*, 356 (26), 2675-2683.

Lusskin, S. I., Pundiak, T. M. & Habib, S. M. (2007). Perinatal depression: Hiding in plain sight. *Canadian Journal of Psychiatry*, 52 (8), 479-578.

Lyons-Ruth, K., Wolfe, R. & Lyubchik, A. (2000). Depression and the parenting of young children: Making the case for early preventive mental health services. *Harvard Review of Psychiatry*, 8 (3), 148-153.

Mazzeo, S. E., Slof-Op't Landt, M. C., Jones, I. et al. (2006). Associations among postpartum depression, eating disorders, and perfectionism in a population-based sample of adult women. *International Journal of Eating Disorders*, 39 (3), 202-211.

McKay, M., Davis, M. & Fanning, P. (1995). *Messages: The communication skills book* (2nd ed.). Oakland: New Harbinger Publications, Inc.

McLeod, J. D. & Kessler, R. C. (1990). Socioeconomic status differences in vulnerability to undesirable life events. *Journal of Health & Social Behavior*, 31 (2), 162-172.

Miller, L. J. (1994). Use of electroconvulsive therapy during pregnancy. *Hospital and Community Psychiatry*, 45 (5), 444-450.

Mischoulon, D. & Fava, M. (2002) Role of S-adenosyl-L-methionine in the treatment of depression: A review of the evidence. *American Journal of Clinical Nutrition*, 76 (5), 1158s–1161s[

Mischoulon, D. & Fava, M. (2000) Docosahexanoic acid and omega-3 fatty acids in depression. *Psychiatric Clinics of North America*, 23 (4), 785-794.

Misri, S. K. (2002). *Shouldn't I be happy? Emotional problems of pregnant and postpartum women.* New York: Free Press.

Misri, S. K. (2005). *Pregnancy blues: What every woman needs to know about depression during pregnancy.* New York: Random House.

Misri, S. & Kendrick, K. (2007). Treatment of perinatal mood and anxiety disorders: A review. *The Canadian Journal of Psychiatry*, 52 (8), 489-498.

Misri, S. & Kostaras, X. (2002). Benefits and risks to mother and infant of drug treatment for postnatal depression. *Drug Safety*, 25 (13), 903-911.

Misri, S., Kostaras, X., Fox, D. et al. (2000). The impact of partner support in the treatment of postpartum depression. *Canadian Journal of Psychiatry*, 45 (6), 554-558.

Misir, S., Oberlander, T. F., Fairbrother, N. et al. (2004). Relation between prenatal maternal mood and anxiety and neonatal health. *Canadian Journal of Psychiatry*, 49, 684-689.

Misri, S. & Sivertz, K. (1991). Tricyclic drugs in pregnancy and lactation: A preliminary report. *International Journal of Psychiatry in Medicine*, 21 (2), 157-171.

Moehler, E., Brunner, R., Wiebel, A. et al. (2006). Maternal depressive symptoms in the postnatal period are associated with long-term impairment of mother-child bonding. *Archives of Women's Mental Health*, 9, 273-278.

Monti, F., Agostini, F., Fagandini, P. et al. (2008). Depressive symptoms during late pregnancy and early parenthood following assisted reproductive technology. *Journal of Perinatal Medicine*, 36, 425–432.

Munk-Olsen, T., Laursen, T.M., Pederson, C.B., et al. (2007). Family and partner psychopathology and the risk of postpartum mental disorders. *Journal of Clinical Psychiatry*, 68 (12), 1947-1953.

Munk-Olsen, T. et al. (2006). New parents and mental disorders: A population-based register study. *Journal of the American Medical Association*, 296, 2582-2589.

Nemets, B., Stahl, Z. & Belmaker, R. H. (2004). Addition of omega-3 fatty acid to maintenance medication treatment for recurrent unipolar depressive disorder. *American Journal of Psychiatry*, 159 (3), 477-449.

Newport, D. J., Hostetter, A., Arnold, A. et al. (2002). The treatment of postpartum depression: Minimizing infant exposures. *Journal of Clinical Psychiatry*, 7, 31-44.

Newport, D. J. et al. (2007). Atypical antipsychotic administration during late pregnancy: Placental passage and obstetrical outcomes. *American Journal of Psychiatry*, 164, 1214-1220.

Nonacs, R. (2006). *A deeper shade of blue: A woman's guide to recognizing and treating depression in her childbearing years.* New York: Simon & Schuster.

Nonacs, R. & Cohen, L. (2003). Assessment and treatment of depression during pregnancy: An update. *Psychiatric Clinics of North America*, 26 (3), 547-562.

Nonacs, R. M., Soares, C. N., Viguera, A. C. et al. (2005). Bupropion SR for the treatment of postpartum depression: A pilot study. *International Journal of Neuropsychopharmacology*, 8, 445-449.

Nulman, I. & Koran, G. (1996). The safety of fluoxetine during pregnancy and lactation. *Teratology*, 53, 304-308.

Nulman, I., Rovet, J., Stewart, D. et al. (1997). Neurodevelopment of children exposed in utero to antidepressant drugs. *New England Journal of Medicine*, 336, 258-262.

Nurnberg, H. G. (2008). Use of sildenafil associated with improvement in antidepressant-related sexual dysfunction in women. *Journal of the American Medical Association*, 300 (4), 395-404.

Oberlander, T. F., Fitzgerald, R. N., Kostaras, X. et al. (2004). Pharmacologic factors associated with transient neonatal symptoms following prenatal psychotropic medication exposure. *Journal of Clinical Psychiatry*, 65, 230-237.

O'Hara, M. W., Rehm, L. P. & Campbell, S. B. (1983). Postpartum depression: A role for social network and life stress variables. *Journal of Nervous and Mental Disorders*, 171, 336-341

O'Hara, M. W., Stuart, S., Gorman, L. L. et al. (2000). Efficacy of interpersonal psychotherapy for postpartum depression. *Archives of General Psychiatry*, 57 (11), 1039-1045.

O'Leary, J. (2004). Grief and its impact on prenatal attachment in the subsequent pregnancy. *Archives of Women's Mental Health*, 7 (1), 7-18.

Olson, A. L., Dietrich, A. J., Prazar, G. et al. (2006). Brief maternal depression screening at well-child visits. *Pediatrics*, 118 (1), 207-216.

Orr, S. T. et al. (2007). Maternal prenatal pregnancy-related anxiety and spontaneous preterm birth in Baltimore, Maryland. *Psychosomatic Medicine*, 69, 566-570.

Patuszak, A., Schick-Boschetto, B., Zuber, C. et al. (1993). Pregnancy outcome following first-trimester exposure to fluoxetine (Prozac). *JAMA*, 269 (17), 2246-2248.

Patton, S. W., Misri, S., Corral, M. R. et al. (2002). Antipsychotic medication during pregnancy and lactation in women with schizophrenia: Evaluating the risk. *Canadian Journal of Psychiatry*, 47 (1), 959-965.

Payne, J. L. (2007). Antidepressant use in the postpartum period: Practical considerations. *American Journal of Psychiatry*, 164 (9), 1329-1332.

Pearlstein, T. B., Zlotnick, C., Battle, C. L. et al. (2006). Patient choice of treatment for postpartum depression: A pilot study. *Archive of Women's Mental Health*, 9, 303-308.

Potts, A. L., Young, K. L., Carter, B. S. et al. (2007). Necrotizing enterocolitis associated with in utero and breast milk exposure to the selective serotonin reuptake inhibitor, escitalopram. *Journal of Perinatology*, 27, 120-122.

Puryear, L. J. (2007). *Understanding your moods when you're expecting: Emotions, mental health, and happiness—before, during, and after pregnancy.* New York: Houghton Mifflin Company.

Ramakrishnan, K. & Scheid, D. C. (2007). Treatment options for insomnia. *American Family Physician*, 76, 517-528.

Repke, J. T. & Berger, N. G. (1984). Electroconvulsive therapy in pregnancy. *Obstetrics and Gynecology*, 63 (suppl.), 39S-40S.

Rippens, J. R., Brawarsky, P., Jackson, R. A. et al. (2006). Association of breastfeeding with maternal depressive symptoms. *Journal of Women's Health*, 15 (6), 754-762.

Roberts, S. L., Bushnell, J. A., Collings, S. C. et al. (2006). Psychological health of men with partners who have post-partum depression. *Australian and New Zealand Journal of Psychiatry*, 40, 704-711.

Robertson, E., Grace, S., Wallington, T. et al. (2004). Antenatal risk factors for postpartum depression: A synthesis of recent literature, *General Hospital Psychiatry*, 26 (4), 289-295.

Robertson, E., Jones, I., Haque, S. et al. (2005). Risk of puerperal and non-puerperal recurrence of illness following bipolar affective puerperal (postpartum) psychosis. *British Journal of Psychiatry*, 186, 258-259.

Ross, L. E. & McLean, L. M. (2006). Anxiety disorders during pregnancy and the postpartum period: A systematic review. *Journal of Clinical Psychiatry*, 67 (8), 1285-1298.

Ross, L. E., Murray, B. J. & Steiner, M. (2005) Sleep and perinatal mood disorders: A critical review. *Journal of Psychiatry & Neuroscience*, 30 (4), 247-256.

Ross, L. E., Steele, L., Goldfinger, C. et al. (2006). Perinatal depressive symptomatology among lesbian and bisexual women. *Archives of Women's Mental Health*, 10, 53-59.

Ross, L. E., Steele, L. & Sapiro, B. (2005). Perceptions of predisposing and protective factors for perinatal depression in same-sex parents. *Journal of Midwifery & Women's Health*, 50 (6), 65-70.

Rubin, E. T., Lee, A. & Ito, S. (2004). When breastfeeding mothers need CNS-acting drugs. *Canadian Journal of Clinical Pharmacology*, 11 (2), 257-266.

Seeman, M. V. (1997). Psychopathology in women and men: Focus on female hormones. *American Journal of Psychiatry*, 154 (12), 1641-1647.

Shapiro, A. F., Gottman, J. M. & Carrere, S. (2000). The baby and the marriage: Identifying factors that buffer against decline in marital satisfaction after the first baby arrives. *Journal of Family Psychology*, 14 (1), 59-70.

Shaw, E. & Kaczorowski, J. (2007). Postpartum care—what's new? *Current Opinion in Obstetrics and Gynecology*, 19, 561-567.

Sit, D. K., Perel J. M., Helsel, J. C. & Wisner, K. L. (2008). Changes in antidepressant metabolism and dosing across pregnancy and early postpartum. *Journal of Clinical Psychiatry*, 69 (4), 652-658.

Sloan, E. P. (2008). Sleep disruption during pregnancy. *Sleep Medicine Clinics*, 3, 73-80.

Spinelli, M. (1997). Interpersonal psychotherapy for depressed antepartum women: A pilot study. *American Journal of Psychiatry*, 154, 1028-1030.

Spinelli, M. G. (2004). Maternal infanticide associated with mental illness: Prevention and the promise of saved lives. *American Journal of Psychiatry*, 161 (9), 1548-1557.

Stapleton, C. (2008). *A promising treatment for depression.* New York: New York Times Syndicate.

Stern, D. (1985). *The interpersonal world of the infant.* New York: Basic Books.

Stewart, D. E., Gagnon, A., Saucier, J. F. et al. (2008). Postpartum depression symptoms in newcomers. *The Canadian Journal of Psychiatry*, 53 (2), 121-124.

Stowe, Z. N. (2007). The use of mood stabilizers during breast-feeding. *Journal of Clinical Psychiatry*, 68 (suppl. 9), 22-28.

Stowe, Z. N., Casarella, J., Landrey, J. et al. (1995). Sertraline in the treatment of women with postpartum major depression. *Depression*, 3, 49-55.

Stowe, Z. N., Cohen, L. S., Hostetter, A. et al. (2000). Paroxetine in human breast milk and nursing infants. *American Journal of Psychiatry*, 157 (2), 185-189.

Stowe, Z. N., Owens, M. J., Landry, J. C. et al. (1997) Sertraline and desmethylsertraline in human breast milk and nursing infants. *American Journal of Psychiatry*, 154, 1255-1260.

Suri, R., Altshuler, L., Hendrick, V. et al. (2004). The impact of depression and fluoxetine treatment on obstetrical outcome. *Archives of Women's Mental Health*, 7 (3), 193-200.

Suri, R. et al. (2007). Effects of antenatal depression and antidepressant treatment on gestational age at birth and risk of preterm birth. *American Journal of Psychiatry*, 164, 1206–1213.

Susman, V. L. & Katz, J. L. (1988) Weaning and depression: Another postpartum complication. *The American Journal of Psychiatry*, 145 (4), 498-501.

Sutter-Dallay, A. L., Murray, L., Glatigny-Dallay, E. et al. (2003). Newborn behavior and risk of postnatal depression in the mother. *Infancy*, 4 (4), 589-602.

Swain, A. M., O'Hara, M. W., Starr, K. R. et al. (1997). A prospective study of sleep, mood, and cognitive function in postpartum and nonpostpartum women. *Obstetrics & Gynecology*, 90 (3), 381-386.

Swinson, R. P. (2006). Clinical practice guidelines: Management of anxiety disorders. *Canadian Journal of Psychiatry*, 51 (suppl. 2), 1S-92S.

Thase, M. E. (2006). Preventing relapse and recurrence of depression: A brief review of therapeutic options. *CNS Spectrums*, 11 (12 suppl. 15), 12-21.

Venis, J. A. & McCloskey, S. (2007). *Postpartum depression demystified: An essential guide to understanding and overcoming the most common complication after childbirth.* New York: Marlowe and Company.

Verhaak, C. M., Smeenk, J. M., van Minnen, A. et al. (2005). A longitudinal, prospective study on emotional adjustment before, during, and after consecutive fertility treatment cycles. *Human Repro-duction*, 20 (8), 2253–2260.

Viguera, A. C., Cohen, L. S., Baldessarini, R. J. et al. (2002). Managing bipolar disorder during pregnancy: Weighing the risks and benefits. *Canadian Journal of Psychiatry*, 47, 426–436.

Viguera, A. C., Cohen, L. S., Bouf-fard, S. et al. (2002) Reproductive decisions by women with bipo-lar disorder after prepregnancy psychiatric consultation. *American Journal of Psychiatry*, 159 (12), 2102–2104.

Viguera, A. C., Newport, D. J., Ritchie, J. et al. (2007). Lithium in breast milk and nursing infants: Clinical implications. *American Journal of Psychiatry*, 164 (2), 342–345.

Viguera, A. C., Nonacs, R., Cohen, L. S. et al. (2000) Risk of recurrence of bipolar disorder in pregnancy and nonpregnant women after dis-continuing lithium maintenance. *American Journal of Psychiatry*, 157 (2), 179–184.

Viguera, A. C., Whitfield, T., Bald-essarini, R. J. et al. (2007). Risk of recurrence in women with bipolar disorder during pregnancy: Pro-spective study of mood stabilizer discontinuation. *American Journal of Psychiatry*, 164 (12), 1817–1824.

Walker, L. O. (2007). Managing excessive weight gain during preg-nancy and the postpartum period. *Journal of Obstetric, Gynecologic & Neonatal Nursing*, 36, 490–500.

Ward, S. & Wisner, K. L. (2007). Collaborative management of women with bipolar disorder dur-ing pregnancy and postpartum: Pharmacologic considerations. *Journal of Midwifery & Women's Health*, 52, 3–13.

Warner, C. H., Bobo, W., Warner, C. et al. (2006). Antidepressant dis-continuation syndrome. *American Family Physician*, 74, 449–457.

WebMD. (2008). *SSRIs: Myths and facts about antidepressants*. http://www.webmd.com/depression/ssris-myths-and-facts-about-antidepressants?page=2

Weissman, A. M., Levy, B. T., Hartz, A. J. et al. (2004). Pooled analysis of antidepressant levels in lactating mothers, breast milk, and nursing infants. *American Journal of Psychiatry*, 161 (6), 1066–1078.

Weissman, M. M. (2007). Recent non-medication trials of interper-sonal psychotherapy for depres-sion. *The International Journal of Neuropsychopharmacology*, 10, 117–122.

Wenzel, A., Haugen, E. N., Jackson, L. C. et al. (2005). Anxiety symp-toms and disorders at eight weeks postpartum. *Journal of Anxiety Disorders*, 19 (3), 295–311.

Wisner, K. L., Chambers, C. & Sit, D. K. Y. (2006). Postpartum depression: A major public health problem. *Journal of the American Medical Association*, 296 (21), 2616-2618.

Wisner, K. L., Gelenberg, A. J., Leonard, H. et al. (1999). Pharmacologic treatment of depression during pregnancy. *JAMA*, 282 (13), 1264-1969.

Wisner, K. L., Parry, B. L. & Piontek, C. M. (2002). Postpartum depression. *New England Journal of Medicine*, 347 (3), 194-199.

Wisner, K. L., Peindl, K. S., Gigliotti, T. et al. (1999). Obsessions and compulsions in women with postpartum depression. *Journal of Clinical Psychiatry*, 60 (3), 176-810.

Wisner, K. L., Perel, J. & Blumer, J. (1998) Serum sertraline and N-desmethylsertraline levels in breastfeeding mother-infant pairs. *American Journal of Psychiatry*, 155, 690–692

Wisner, K. L., Perel, J. M., Peindl, K. S. et al. (2004). Prevention of postpartum depression: A pilot randomized clinical trial. *American Journal of Psychiatry*, 161 (7), 1290-1292.

Wisner, P. (2001). Prevention of recurrent postpartum major depression. *Hospital and Community Psychiatry*, 62 (2), 82-86.

Wolfson, A. R., Crowley, S. J., Anwer, U. et al. (2003). Changes in sleep patterns and depressive symptoms in first-time mothers: Last trimester to 1-year postpartum. *Behavioral Sleep Medicine*, 1 (1), 54-67.

Yonkers, K. A., Lin, H., Howell, H. B., et al. (2008) Pharmacologic treatment of postpartum women with new-onset major depressive disorder: A randomized control trial with paroxetine. *Journal of Clinical Psychiatry*, 69 (4), 659-665.

Yonkers, K. A., Wisner, K. L., Stowe, Z. et al. (2004) Management of bipolar disorder during pregnancy and the postpartum period. *American Journal of Psychiatry*, 161 (4), 608-620.

Zelkowitz, P. & Milet, T. H. (2001). The course of postpartum psychiatric disorders in women and their partners. *Journal of Nervous and Mental Disorders*, 189 (9), 575-582.

Zeskind, P. & Stephens, L. (2004). Maternal selective serotonin reuptake inhibitor use during pregnancy and newborn neurobehavior. *Pediatrics*, 113 (2), 368-375.

Index